Acupressure

for

Lovers

Acupressure for Lovers

Secrets of Touch for Increasing Intimacy

Michael Reed Gach, Ph.D.

BANTAM BOOKS

NEW YORK • TORONTO • LONDON • SYDNEY • AUCKLAND

Acupressure for Lovers
A Bantam Book/February 1997
The BANTAM NEW AGE BOOKS logo is a registered trademark of Bantam Doubleday Dell Publishing Group, Inc.

Library of Congress Cataloging-in-Publication Data
Gach, Michael Reed.
Acupressure for lovers : secrets of touch for increasing intimacy / Michael Reed Gach.
    p. cm.
ISBN 0-553-37401-X (pbk.)
1. Sex instruction. 2. Acupressure points.
I. Title.
HQ31.G12 1997
613.9′07—dc20   96-20841 CIP

Bantam Books are published by Bantam Books, a division of Bantam Doubleday Dell Publishing Group, Inc. Its trademark, consisting of the words "Bantam Books" and the portrayal of a rooster, is registered in the U.S. Patent and Trademark Office and in other countries. Marca Registrada. Bantam Books, 1540 Broadway, New York, New York 10036.

Printed in the United States of America
BP 0 9 8 7 6 5 4 3 2 1

DEDICATION

To all couples:

May this book deepen

your intimacy and pleasure.

May it provide new ways

to open your heart and connect with your partner,

enhancing your love and lives together.

Sharing your innermost selves passionately

in a sexual relationship

is a sacred journey.

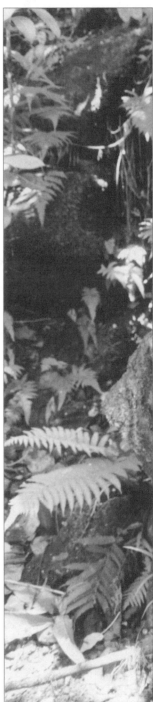

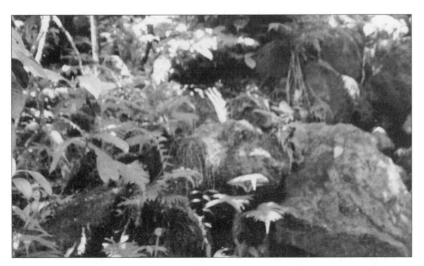

CONTENTS

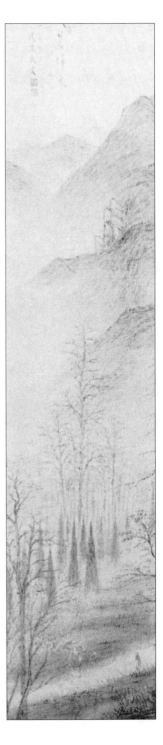

Introduction

Two of my closest friends, Gail and Scott, who took my acupressure training several years ago, recently returned to my school to take a refresher course. Gail and Scott loved each other very much, but their sex life had grown stale. The first six months of their relationship had been filled with intimacy and a powerful, erotic alchemy, but ten years later, both Gail and Scott had become too tired to make love, their lives ruled more by work than intimacy. Sex became "sort of mechanical."

Gail and Scott have always been comfortable sharing their feelings with me. When I told them about the couples' exercises that I was developing for a new book on acupressure for lovers, they were both eager to explore the erotic movements and give me feedback about how they worked. Six weeks after I had suggested a series of exercises, they reported back to me that their sexual vitality had increased significantly. Each new position and way of touching had opened up a new dimension to their togetherness.

Scott told me that although he knew the importance of foreplay, when Gail and he made love he always had a strong desire to skip it. Often he would merely try to prepare Gail for intercourse by stimulating her genitals with his fingers. The more accustomed he became to giving Gail this kind of pre-intercourse stimulation and to expecting her to respond to it, the more blocked their sexual relationship had become. He admitted that he was feeling extremely frustrated with her. Since they had started to practice the couples' acupressure exercises, however, Scott said that his feelings of intimacy and sexual connection with Gail had begun to grow again.

Gail also attested that they felt a renewal of their initial magnetic attraction. One weekend they were sitting naked in bed together, touching each other playfully. Gail was sitting in Scott's lap facing him with her legs wrapped around him, stimulating acupressure points in his buttocks with her heels, and holding his neck with her fingers. Scott's arms were wrapped around her, holding points in her lower back. They rocked back and forth in slow motion, breathing together. As they held the points, Gail felt a tremendous flow

We shall not cease from exploration and the end of all our exploring will be to arrive where we started and know the place for the first time.

—T. S. Eliot

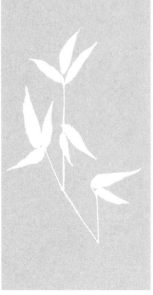

circulating throughout her body. Both were aware of pleasure all over their skin as they embraced and slid against each other.

The acupressure for lovers experience was exhilarating for both of them. Scott was especially pleased to have broken out of his habit of targeting only one area of Gail's body. They had begun to relax with each other, relax their expectations of each other, and undergo powerful feelings of transcendence that were difficult to express in words.

ENHANCING YOUR LOVE LIFE THROUGH ACUPRESSURE

This book provides a wide menu of intimacy-building and health-building exercises for couples. You will learn ways to explore your partner's body and mind through embraces, stretches, movements, and presence. You will also learn how to care for each other physically and emotionally through the power of touch. Touching and holding significant points on the body relieves pain, increases erotic energy, promotes healing, and fosters relaxation. Acupressure for lovers can deepen your bonds of trust and compassion. By practicing the acupressure exercises in the following chapters and becoming more aware of the powerful energy in the human body, you can enhance your health and your love relationship.

I have practiced and taught acupressure therapy for more than twenty years. During this time, I have had numerous powerful healing experiences that provided me profound insights into how the body works. Acupressure can intensify physical pleasure and sexual energies that open to transcendent experiences. It also transforms sexual energy to enhance spiritual healing and increase intimacy.

It's difficult to be intimate when either you or your partner is preoccupied, tense, or upset. When your partner comes home a bundle of nerves, relaxing physical contact can ease the stress more quickly than talking. If your partner is willing to lie down and have you work on his or her shoulders and back, a complete change of mood can occur within twenty minutes.

There are special ways to use acupressure points on your partner to create intimacy and improve the chemistry of a love relationship. These points are the same as those used in acupuncture, but instead of using needles, couples can energize these vital points through the power of touch. This book will show you many different ways to arouse and satisfy your partner by activating these points on various parts of the body.

When your partner gives you a big, satisfying hug, specific acupressure points are being stimulated. Each point, depending upon how it is touched, has a unique effect. Some points relax us while others arouse us, opening us up to intense, pleasurable sensations.

Just as we instinctively touch tense or aching points on our own bodies, or knead a pulled muscle to help relieve the pain, we also often rub or massage areas of our body that just feel good to touch. And we use these same instincts when we touch our partners in areas that feel good.

Be glad of life! Because it gives you the chance to love and work; to play and look up at the stars.

—Henry Van Dyke

USING THIS BOOK EFFECTIVELY

Acupressure for Lovers is designed primarily for romantically involved couples to use in privacy to develop their sacred sexuality and increase their intimacy. These acupressure point references and techniques are not intended to be used professionally by acupressurists, massage therapists, or other professional bodyworkers.

Even though the title, *Acupressure for Lovers,* seems to exclude all but intimate couples from participating in the use of this book, friends, coworkers, and even solitary individuals can also use many of the bodywork, acupressure, and stretching exercises in this book. You can learn new ways to reach out to others and offer touch in a safe, nonsexual, healing context.

Although you may read this book from cover to cover, you do not need to do so to derive benefit from it. It has been organized in a way that will help you become progressively more intimate and sexual with your mate, but you may also pick and choose from among the different chapters, as you would from a buffet that offers a variety of delicious courses and flavors, for developing intimacy in your relationship.

For Couples

The healing touch of the acupressure techniques in this book can help you more fully appreciate and physically enjoy your own and your lover's body. The respectful, healing touch of the stretches, bodywork, and couples' exercises can cultivate the friendship within your romantic relationship and also lead to mutually satisfying sexual interactions by having new and playful ways of making love. You will feel good knowing that you are giving hands-on care to a loved one and becoming a more creative and understanding sexual partner.

In the beginning, your partner may be skeptical or resistant to trying out new sexual activities. If you anticipate a reaction of this sort, I recommend that before trying some of the more advanced techniques in the book, you introduce nonthreatening activities such as the shoulder massage in Chapter 5 or the mutual foot massage in Chapter 8. Simply try a few of the points and suggestions in Chapter 4 on Building Intimacy and Chapter 5 on Preparing for Love that you think your partner might enjoy. After you find a few hands-on techniques that your lover really likes, incorporate these acupressure techniques into your lovemaking. Once your partner is open to exploring these activities with you, the following guidelines become helpful.

For Daily Practice

While establishing a regular hour-long acupressure routine may be unrealistic, you may be able to work on each other for ten to twenty minutes a day. After reviewing the acupressure love positions in Chapter 8, choose a routine you like the most to use as a daily morning or evening practice. In addition to these exercises, I suggest regularly practicing any of the following activities:

• Touch your partner as he or she is waking up. Establish a full-body ritual, wholeheartedly embracing your loved one each morning before you rise.

• Hug your partner several times a day.

• Make contact with your love at mid-day, offering support. Greet each other with eye contact as well as with your bodies.

• Exchange a shoulder and neck massage to greet each other at the end of a busy day.

• Express your love as you lie in bed in the evening, sharing the trouble and beauty the day has brought.

A Weekly Sexual Delight

This book encourages you to commit to deepening your sexual intimacy as a couple. In addition to any spontaneous sexual embraces with your mate, I suggest a weekly sexual practice, setting aside a regular, sacred time to express your love for each other.

Find the best time in your schedule for a weekly date, and take an hour or two to luxuriate in each other's touch. Offer kisses and embraces with sweetness and mutual affection. Each week, consciously prepare a nurturing environment for making love—Chapter 1 details how to create a sacred space. You might include the following activities in your weekly sexual delight:

• Begin with some of the couples' stretches from Chapter 4.

• Choose one of the Thai massage routines from Chapter 11.

• Select one of the Lovemaking Progressions in Chapter 10 to play and express your sexuality.

During Special Times

Planning to share special events with your partner is an important dimension to enriching your lives together. In addition to having a daily intimate practice and a weekly date, you might try the Lovemaking Progressions during special times such as a vacation, retreat, or holiday. Consider these times away from your regular work routine as an opportunity to recommit.

Every couple's life has periods of stress and you can use this book at such times to lift your spirits, enhance your intimacy, and help you be present for your partner in a significant, responsible way.

Lists for Lovers

As you progress through this book, make a list of the stretches, exercises, acupressure points, positions, rituals, and suggestions that you and your partner find most satisfying and helpful. Organize this list into three categories:

1. Short, daily practices you can do in and out of bed. These may be your favorite acupressure points in Chapters 9 and 10 or the Thai Massage and Advanced Couple Work in Chapter 11.

2. Your favorite acupressure love positions from Chapter 8.

3. A Lovemaking Progression from Chapter 10.

List all of the activities you would like to share with your partner. Once you have organized these three lists, buy some colored Post-its

Frequent changes of position become extremely important. It is important that lovemaking loses none of its attractions through thoughtless repetitions and that partners do not become bored with one another.

—Jolan Chang
The Tao of Love and Sex

or tabs from a stationery store. Assign a different color for each of these three categories. For example:

• Yellow tabs can represent daily practices.

• Pink tabs can correspond to your favorite weekly routines.

• Blue tabs can designate the sections of the book you want to use without time constraints, exploring with more depth.

This method can help you to organize your favorite routines according to your needs and lifestyle.

OPEN TO INTIMACY

By developing these conscious practices into sacred rituals you will cultivate deeper intimacy. The nurturing and attention you give your relationship will facilitate your communication and open your hearts. Whether you try a few acupressure points or love positions or share a meal, a massage, or a meditation, it's important that you create spiritual and sexual practices that fit your individual bodies and sensual preferences. Once you become accustomed to the routines you formulate with your lover, your bodies can flow together without having to use this book. Enjoying your favorite points, bodywork, stretches, postures, personal daily routines, and special love rituals will become as natural as breathing.

Chapter 1

ACUPRESSURE GUIDELINES
FOR LOVERS

*A*cupressure can be done by both men and women, both young and old. Exactly why it works is somewhat mysterious, but how to do it is relatively simple and straightforward. This chapter will show you how to stimulate acupressure points, how much pressure to use, how long to hold each point, and most important, how to locate the points. Then we will consider some special ways to make acupressure experiences intimate and rewarding. Finally, this chapter presents six sets of acupressure points that are important for romantic and sexual applications.

ACUPRESSURE AND SEXUALITY

Acupressure is an ancient healing system that was developed over several centuries by Chinese doctors who observed that muscular tension tends to concentrate around certain points in the body. Tension that accumulates and becomes chronic acts like a traffic jam and blocks the free circulation of energy through the body. This blockage sets the stage for stress disorders and sexual problems.

Acupressure releases muscular tension and eliminates the toxins held in the muscle tissue, thereby enabling energy and blood to flow freely. As blood circulation increases, oxygen and other nutrients can nourish more areas of the body, naturally heightening a person's sensuality. When the blood and energy are circulating properly, the person has a greater sense of responsiveness and vibrancy.

Using the same points known to be medically therapeutic, the Chinese people discovered many highly erotic techniques. For instance, exerting firm prolonged pressure into the small indentations

One of the secrets of successful body touching is to make contact from head to toe at as many points as you can. Touching in loving should not be static. Keep your hands flowing over your partner's body; your body responding to the subtle variations as she breathes or moves against you.

—Jolan Chang
The Tao of Love and Sex

of the large triangular bone at the base of the spine (the sacrum) is a technique used clinically to relieve menstrual cramps, labor pains, sciatica, low back pain, and urinary tract disorders. But pressing the acupressure points at the base of the spine stimulates the genital region as well, so that it is often sexually arousing.

In Chinese medicine, acupressure points are considered gateways for human electrical energy. This energy, often referred to as the life force (in Japanese *ki*, in Chinese *chi*) moves throughout the body along pathways called meridians. A clear flow of energy through the meridians is the key to radiant health, eroticism, and intimacy. Acupressure points are the junctures of these energy pathways.

Holding acupressure points for more than a minute or so causes the body to release neurochemicals called endorphins, the body's natural painkillers. The release of endorphins can create a euphoric "natural high" and encourage relaxation as well as magnetism and intimacy. In addition to acupressure, meditation, aerobic exercise, and lovemaking all stimulate the release of endorphins.

How to Do Acupressure

You can practice acupressure with a partner in any number of ways. You can press and hold the points while you are hugging, whether as an affectionate greeting or while making love. You may incorporate acupressure into a shoulder and neck massage to relax your partner after a stressful day. You may press and hold points to relieve a headache or help your partner get to sleep at night. There are numerous ways to stimulate the points: you can caress, kiss, lick, suck, and knead them as well as rub them. Often, however, the most powerful stimulation is simply to hold the point firmly.

Acupressure's healing touch is safe to do on yourself and others—even if you have never done it before—as long as you follow the instructions and pay attention to the cautions. It is noninvasive and produces no druglike side effects. Since the only equipment you need is your own two hands, you can practice acupressure anytime, anywhere.

To help you locate the points, the illustrations at the end of each couple's exercise show you the major acupressure points stimulated in that exercise. In addition, Appendix A lists some of the major acupressure points for relieving common ailments and catalogs their many health benefits. For more detailed health information, refer to my previous book, *Acupressure's Potent Points.* If you or your partner has any of these ailments, you may wish to hold some of these points during the intimacy exercises.

NAMES OF POINTS

Each of the 365 acupressure points has been poetically named, based on ancient sources of traditional Chinese medicine. Often the name provides insight into the point's location or its benefits. For instance, holding the point called Rushing Door, located in the groin, can open a rush of circulation into the genitals and legs. It is sexually arousing as well as good for relieving cold feet.

In the illustrations in this book, however, the points are labeled by number. These point reference numbers follow standard abbreviations used by professional acupressurists and acupuncturists. The point labeled Sp 6, for instance, is the sixth point on the spleen meridian. Lovers do not need to know or try to remember these point reference numbers to enjoy the many benefits of acupressure.

HOW TO FIND THE POINTS

Most acupressure points can be located by using major anatomical landmarks, such as bone indentations and protrusions. For instance, the point called Facial Beauty (St 3) is located directly below the center of the eye, a half-inch outside the nose, in a slight indentation underneath the cheekbone. This point is usually quite sensitive to firm pressure.

Avoid pressing directly on bones unless you feel an indentation. For instance, when pressing the sacrum at the base of the spine, press gently into the indentations in the hollow of the bone.

While some points lie near bony landmarks, others are located underneath major muscle groups. To find these points, feel for a muscular cord or a slight depression between the tendons and muscles. Once you have found a muscular cord, press on it slowly and directly.

Acupressure points often feel sore upon pressure. Ask your partner to alert you to any tenderness. The tenderness is a signal that you have found a point's exact location, but you must apply the pressure slowly and carefully so that you don't hurt your partner. Sometimes points can become extremely sore; at other times, they may not get

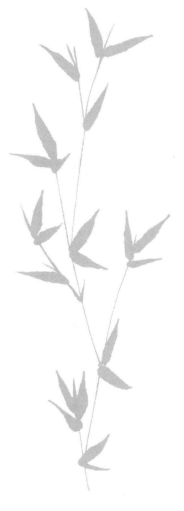

sore at all, due to the hardened chronic tension covering them. If you find increasing or extreme sensitivity or pain at a point, gradually decrease the pressure until you achieve a balance between pain and pleasure.

HOW TO TOUCH THE POINTS

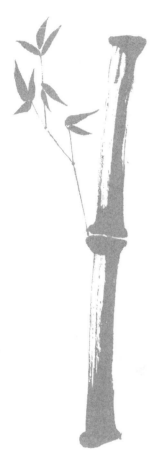

To touch a point, apply finger pressure gradually, aiming into the center of the body part. Hold your finger or hand perpendicular to the surface of the skin. Any pull on the skin means that the angle of pressure is incorrect. Consciously direct your finger pressure into the center of the body part being worked on. Your nails should be short.

Always remember to apply pressure gradually. The more slowly you apply pressure to the point, the more effective your fingers will be. Applying pressure gradually allows the tissues to respond, promotes healing, and encourages your partner to feel connected to you.

Use your whole body to apply finger pressure, carefully leaning your weight into the point. It is important to do this even if you are using your hand to grasp or squeeze the point. Gradually lean your body toward your partner, staying on the point, and ask your partner to take several long, slow, deep breaths. Try to breathe in unison, following your partner's lead.

Hold each point for 1 to 5 minutes as you breathe deeply together. The tighter or more painful a point is, the longer you should hold it, but limit the pressure to 5 minutes maximum. While holding a point, adjust the pressure so that you do not hurt your partner. Feel for a pulse. A clear regular pulse indicates increased circulation, so pay attention to its strength and quality. If the pulse is faint or throbbing, continue to hold the point. When it becomes regular and balanced, slowly decrease your finger pressure, ending with a light loving touch.

HOW MUCH PRESSURE TO APPLY

Every body and every area of the body will require a different amount of pressure. Some areas of the body tend to be sensitive, such as the calves, the backs of the knees, the face, and the genitals. Many people like deeper pressure in the areas of the back, buttocks, and neck. But start off gently.

The right amount of pressure will vary greatly depending upon how physically fit the person's body is. A healthy, more muscularly developed body will require more pressure. For a person who gets little daily exercise or tends to be sensitive, use a light touch instead. If a person has a medical condition, disease, or weakness, consult a qualified health professional who has experience in acupressure. For most such people, a light touch is safe and appropriate.

Generally, men's bodies tend to be more muscular than women's and thus need deeper pressure. Since we often give what we want to receive, however, men typically massage women's bodies firmly and deeply, the way men like to be massaged. A woman on the receiving end of this kind of treatment might think to herself, "I can't wait until he stops gouging me, so I can show him what really feels good." When she massages him, she may apply the pressure more gently and slowly, with sensitivity and care. Meanwhile, he'll be thinking, "I wish she'd go deeper. Next time I work on her, I'll show her how to do it." To avoid this common scenario, partners need to communicate clearly and express their particular needs.

Explore innovative ways of holding each other's points. To discover what your partner prefers, try light and then deeper ways of touching points. You may at first try steady pressure with your fingertips, then learn that your partner likes a repeated, staccatolike pressure or a slight circular movement. If your partner wants deeper pressure, you may try using your knuckles, or the whole palm of your hand.

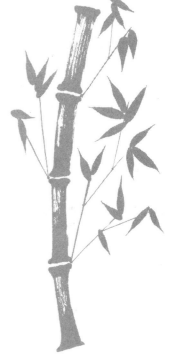

The stimulation of one point can send a healing message to other parts of the body, so that each acupressure point has different applications for lovers. Pressing the points in the groin can not only increase genital pleasure and arousal but also increase circulation in the legs and thereby benefit cold feet. One point can act as a gateway to many parts of the body. Thus, in the following chapters you will find the same acupressure points used for a variety of purposes.

Most important for lovers, as you use acupressure, promise yourself and each other that you will remain present in the moment. Try not to let your mind wander, for it is only by paying close attention to the responses of your and your partner's bodies that you will achieve full emotional, erotic, and spiritual intimacy.

SPECIAL SUGGESTIONS FOR LOVERS

The following suggestions for successful acupressure experiences invite you to make use of your breath, your capacity to notice sensation, your inner sensitivity to touch, and your capacities to move and communicate. As you tap each of these resources, imagine you are in an erotic playground. Relax and explore your partner, and be explored by the person you trust more than anyone in the world.

Chinese erotic terms conjure up all sorts of images in the minds of the participants, and this imagery greatly enhances the ambiance of sexual intercouse.

—Daniel P. Reid
The Tao of Health, Sex, and Longevity

Set the Scene

First, create a special environment for giving and receiving acupressure. Having a special private place is a key for cultivating intimacy. It may well be your bedroom.

Make sure the place is comfortably warm, because your body may tense up if you're cold. Don't cover yourself with a blanket; this can inhibit your movements, especially during the positions and Lovemaking Progressions in Chapters 9 and 10. You may wear comfortable, light, natural fiber clothing, or you may wear nothing at all. If you are naked, make sure the room is toasty warm.

Have plenty of pillows around, and a clean flat sheet to sit or lie on, whether it is on the floor or on the bed.

Lighting is important for creating a romantic environment. Dim the lights, or better yet, light a few candles and place them around the room. Candlelight's soft glow enhances skin tones. If you have no candles, place a scarf over a lamp for subdued lighting—but be sure it is far enough away from the bulb that it doesn't create a fire hazard. You may also want to play relaxing, quiet music.

Create sacred time—an hour each day, an afternoon each week, or a weekend each month—to be alone together, to respond to each other in a natural, unpressured, and unscheduled way. Come without expectations or an agenda. Nothing is "supposed" to happen; the only goal is to be present in each other's company.

Breathe Deeply

Breathing is the most important key to relieving aches and pains, tension, and anxiety. The way you breathe is a barometer of your mind and emotions, including your love relationship. When your breathing is shallow, you may easily become irritable, inaccessible, depressed, or fatigued. On the other hand, slow deep breathing can free the emotions necessary to deepen intimacy. Increasing the capacity of your breath—making it long, deep, and smooth—can provide an abundance of energy, greater clarity, and full awareness. You will feel better about yourself and your relationship.

Deep-belly breathing is a profound tool for couples who want to heighten their experience of lovemaking. Visualize each breath as having four parts:

- a slow, deep inhalation

- several seconds with the breath held

- an even slower exhalation

- a momentary pause before beginning the next inhalation

When your breathing is long and deep, your body cells become fully nourished and oxygenated, enabling you to feel more. Whatever feelings or body sensations surface, continue to breathe deeply and be present with your partner. Simply listen and breathe without rationalizing or judging. By being in the present moment while you breathe, touch, and hold each other, you can share the innermost parts of yourselves—without uttering a word! This is how deep breathing nurtures sexual intimacy.

While practicing the exercises in this book with your partner, remember to take full, slow, complete breaths together. By nourishing your bodies with breath, you will generate a greater feeling of well-being in your relationship. The many far-reaching effects of deep conscious breathing include:

- fortifying your sexual reproductive system

- increasing your sensual awareness and pleasures

- enhancing your vital energy, opening your heart to love, and stabilizing your emotional intimacy

- bringing you into the present moment, enabling you to participate fully in an intimate sexual exchange

When correct breathing is practiced, the myriad ailments will not occur. When breathing is depressed or strained, all sorts of diseases will arise. Those who wish to nurture their lives must first learn the correct methods of controlling breath and balancing energy. These breathing methods can cure all ailments great and small.

—Dr. Sun Ssu-Mo
Precious Recipes

Breathing deeply together is one of the most profound ways to cultivate your sexual relationship.

Deep Breathing: Try this couple's breathing exercise while you cuddle in a spooning position, using pillows to support your heads. The partner behind places one arm underneath his or her partner's neck and holds the breastbone or forehead. The other hand holds the lower belly and is free to touch the genitals. Close your eyes and adjust your bodies comfortably, with your feet or ankles touching your partner's.

As you cuddle and breathe deeply together, notice your bodily sensations. Breathe in and out slowly and deeply in synchronization for several minutes. Let go of whatever feelings, memories, or judgments you're holding from the past; let go of whatever anxiety you have about the present or the future. Consciously focus on being in the present moment, feeling your body as you continue to breathe deeply in sync. . . . Ask yourselves what your hearts need. Be with the question and let the answers simply come to you. . . . Whether you drift off to sleep or become sexually charged and aroused, let yourselves go with the flow.

Breath Alternation: Another way to practice couple's breathing is simply to breathe in slowly and deeply as your partner breathes out. After pausing for a few seconds, breathe out as your partner breathes in. Continue to breathe slowly and deeply in this way for several minutes as you focus on loving your partner.

After trying both ways of breathing, choose one pattern that seems most mutually satisfying. Breathing deeply together on a daily basis generates energy for a more vibrant loving couple.

Relax Your Body

The most trustworthy personal information you have comes from your own body. Your body does not lie but provides constant and direct responses to your experiences. The more you pay attention to its signals, including its minutest sensations, the easier it will be to interpret them. Intimacy requires you to be relaxed and yet attuned to the signals of your body. Cultivating body awareness, deep relaxation, and the ability to communicate your body's responses will enable you to be more responsive to each other.

I add my breath

To your breath

That our days may

Be long on the Earth

That the days

Of our people

May be long

That we may

Be one person.

—Translated by
Paula Gunn Allen
Ancient Keres song

Daily stretching, such as yoga, awakens your body's circulation in new ways, and with good results for your love life. Without regular stretching, the body becomes stiff, tense, and easily tired. Everyone must take responsibility for stretching and for maintaining good overall body awareness and health.

As you stretch, tune in to your body. Close your eyes and focus your attention on how each body part feels. Don't force your body into uncomfortable stretching positions, and don't strain it. Let it stretch as far as it wants to go, trusting your judgment and your own limitations. Be flexible; the degree of your stretch at any particular time may vary, depending on many circumstances. Stretch slowly and moderately, so that you feel a small degree of pull but not pain. If you experience pain in a stretch, you are pushing yourself too hard.

Immediately after stretching, practicing the couple's exercises, or using acupressure points, lie down on your back and make yourself comfortable, covering yourself with a blanket or a sheet. The following relaxation meditation can help you relax from your toes to your head. You may want to make a tape recording of these steps, perhaps accompanied by soothing background music.

Close your eyes, take several long, slow, deep breaths, and settle into your body's awareness. . . .

Wiggle your toes and feet, and let them relax. . . . Feel your legs . . . your calves, knees, and thighs relax. . . . Tighten your buttock muscles and let them relax. . . . Feel your sex organs and pelvis relax. . . . Take several more long, deep breaths into your abdominal area, letting your belly relax. . . . Just let yourself relax. . . .

Let your whole back relax. . . . Relax your arms and wrists. . . . Feel each finger relax. . . . Now tell your shoulders and neck to relax. . . . Let your forehead, temples, eyebrows, the bridge of your nose, your eyelids completely relax. . . . Lips, gums, teeth, and throat . . . relax. Move your jaw from side to side, letting it relax. Inhale, taking a slow, deep breath . . . and let yourself go, relaxing as you exhale. . . . Tell all the muscles in back of your eyes to just relax. . . . Relax your eyelids. Once again, inhale deeply. Exhale . . . and totally relax. . . . Continue breathing deeply. . . .

Now, let the inner core of your head relax. . . . Simply feel your whole body being completely supported. . . . With each full deep breath you take, envision your body being held, loved, and cared for by the wise universe. . . . Let yourself go. . . . Just relax. . . .

There is one way of breathing that is shameful and constricted. Then there's another way: a breath of love that takes you all the way to infinity.

—Rumi
Open Secret

Apply a Healing Touch

Conscious touching treats your partner's body as a sacred vessel. Touching with the intention of awakening your partner's pleasure and innermost feelings expands your ability to care for your mate and amplifies the magnetism in your love relationship.

If your partner has a tight muscle or joint pain (not caused by a recent or severe injury), focus your attention on that tense or painful spot by gradually applying finger pressure. Slowly make direct contact with the muscular tightness or pain. Make sure your partner is sitting or lying in a comfortable position with eyes closed. Take long, slow, complete breaths as you coach your partner for 3 to 5 minutes in the following manner:

Inhale slowly and deeply into your abdomen, letting your belly expand. As the air begins to fill your lungs, feel the breath reach into the depths of your belly. Exhale slowly, letting the energy you drew in circulate throughout your body. . . . Continue to focus on breathing into your discomfort, feeling some of the tension or pain release and leave your body each time you exhale.

When you inhale, imagine you are breathing in healing energy and channeling it into the tension or painful spot as you steadily press it. Once the tension or pain subsides, reposition your bodies to embrace comfortably. Concentrate on breathing deeply in synchronicity with each other as you give your partner a full body hug.

THE TOP SIX SETS OF ACUPRESSURE POINTS FOR LOVERS

These acupressure points are those used most frequently in love relationships and will be referred to throughout the book. Familiarize yourself with them. Learn where they are located, their names, and their love-related applications.

Points located close together have similar functions and are grouped together as sets. Conveniently, these points are to be pressed at the same time. For instance, the points on the base of the spine are located so close together that applying pressure with the heel of your hand can stimulate all of them at once. As you read about the points, visualize how it would feel to give and receive acupressure's touch with your partner.

Just as the eyes see light and translate it into an image and the ears hear sounds and translate them into signals, there is a largely unrecognized dimension of human capability that experiences energy more directly than as feelings, attitudes and impressions. For this dimension of human awareness, energy becomes a living current.

—Richard Moss, M.D.
The I That Is We

Rushing Door (Sp 12) and Mansion Cottage (Sp 13)

Located in the center of the groin on both sides, Rushing Door (Sp 12) and Mansion Cottage (Sp 13) are a major gate for energy flow into the genitals and can enhance your partner's sexual pleasure. When these points are opened, energy freely flows through the reproductive system, enabling a wider spectrum of feeling in the area.

Location: Both these points lie in the pelvic area close to the middle of the crease where the leg joins the trunk of the body.

Applications: With your partner lying on his or her back, gently place the heels of your hands on the groin creases on both sides where the thigh joins the trunk of the body. Adjust your hands for your comfort. With your fingertips lightly on the belly, slowly lean the weight of your chest into the Rushing Door points, gradually increasing the pressure.

Ask your partner how much pressure feels right before you lean your full weight into the points. Regulate the amount of pressure so that it is pleasurably intense for him or her. Encourage your partner to breathe deeply into the lower abdomen as you continue to lean into the Rushing Door points for approximately 2 minutes.

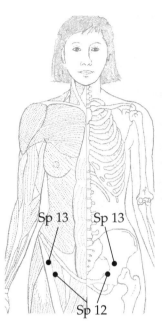

Sea of Vitality (B 23 and B 47)

These points (B 23, B 47) were named after their ability to cultivate both physical and sexual energy. They are the best points to press in the lower back while hugging your partner. A couple of minutes of pressure on the Sea of Vitality points can benefit the kidneys, which store sexual energy and govern the reproductive system. Use these points on a regular basis for enhancing your sexual vitality.

Caution: Do not press on disintegrating disks or fractured or broken bones. For someone with a weak back, a few minutes of stationary light touching instead of pressure can be healing. See your doctor first if you need medical advice.

Location: These points lie on the lower back, between the second and third lumbar vertebrae, 2 and 4 finger-widths away from the spine at waist level, in line with the belly button.

Applications: Hug your partner front-to-front in any position. Place one of your hands over the lower back, with your other hand over that hand for support. Firmly squeeze the ropelike muscular cords on both sides of the lower back, using your fingertips on one side and the heel of your hand on the other, for 1 to 2 minutes.

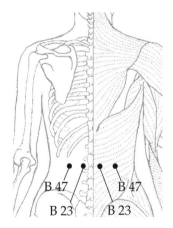

Womb and Vitals (B 27–B 34) *and Sacral Points* (B 48)

These sets of points (B 27–B 34, B 48) increase circulation through the pelvis and nurture a woman's womb. As the name indicates, the Womb and Vitals and Sacral Points strongly benefit the reproductive system. Pressing these points triggers the sacral nerves and thereby stimulates the genitals. You can use these points for arousing your partner and during intercourse itself.

Location: These points lie on the base of the spine in the hollows of the sacrum, the large bony area at the base of the spine. B 48 is located 1 to 2 finger-widths outside the sacrum and midway between the top of the hip bone and the base of the buttocks.

Applications: Try using these arousal points during oral sex and intercourse. Feel for the slight indentations at the base of your partner's spine and firmly hold these hollow areas with your fingertips. As you hug your partner front to front, gradually apply firm pressure to these points. This will bring your pelvises closer, providing stronger stimulation and greater pleasure. One minute of firm pressure on the Womb and Vitals points can significantly increase your partner's sexual pleasure.

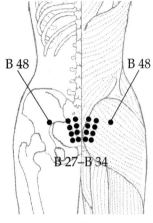

B 48 · B 48 · B 27–B 34

Sacral Points

Inner Meeting (CV 1)

Inner Meeting (CV 1) is an intimate point for enhancing a woman's orgasm and a man's ejaculation. Holding this point with various amounts of finger pressure can generate a deeper intimacy in your sexual life.

Location: At the center of the perineum, midway between the anus and genitals, you will feel a ropy cordlike structure under the surface of the skin. Gradually apply firm pressure directly onto the cord in a hollow area.

Applications: Inner Meeting is a powerful point for building sexual intimacy since it is located in one of the most vulnerable areas of the body. CV 1 can also stimulate the prostate gland and prolong a man's orgasm. (See Increasing a Man's Sexual Pleasure in Chapter 7.)

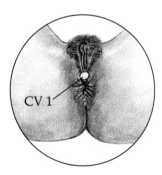

CV 1

Sea of Intimacy (CV 4–CV 6)

These lower abdominal points (CV 4–CV 6) restore, secure, and supplement sexual intimacy. Ancient Chinese sexology considered the Sea of Intimacy to be the center of the human body, because all of the inner meridians that come up from the genital region pass through the area. Applying gradual pressure to these points can release the lower abdominal area, which commonly cramps involuntarily when sexual energies are aroused. The Sea of Intimacy is used to treat a variety of sexual problems, including impotence, premature ejaculation, inhibited sexual desire, and infertility.

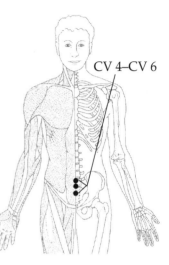

Location: These points are located two, three, and four finger-widths below the navel, on a line between the navel and pubic bone.

Applications: The Sea of Intimacy is an excellent set of points to press either before or during intercourse. If you are on top, place the palms of your hands on your partner's lower abdominal area, gradually applying firm pressure. Encourage your partner to breathe into your hands as you hold firmly for 2 to 3 minutes. Synchronizing your breathing while maintaining eye contact can be an especially powerful and intimate experience. The Sea of Intimacy points can be especially arousing to a woman. (See Chapter 6.)

Sea of Tranquility (CV 17)

Sea of Tranquility (CV 17) is an emotional balancing point that opens and calms the spirit of the heart. When you hug your partner and feel your hearts connect, your breastbones are pressing each other's Sea of Tranquility points. The name Sea of Tranquility refers to the point's calming and relaxing influence.

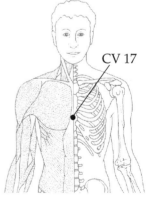

Location: This point lies on the center of the breastbone, four finger-widths up from the base of the bone.

Applications: The Sea of Tranquility has a wide range of uses in a love relationship. Try using this point when your partner is anxious, nervous, or tense. Either hug your partner, or place one hand on the breastbone and your other hand directly behind, on the upper back. With your eyes closed, breathe deeply together for a few minutes.

While being sexual together with your partner's shirt off, kiss and suck the Sea of Tranquility point for a minute or two. Front-to-front intercourse presses this point naturally. After intercourse, hold this point on each other, placing the palms of your hands between the shoulder blades while you breathe deeply together.

BEYOND THE ORGASM

Acupressure for Lovers aims to inspire your whole body, not just the genitals. Sexuality is not limited to intercourse and orgasm; it involves your mind, body, and spirit. When you practice acupressure with your partner, you stimulate all parts of your bodies. As your feet are pressed, your buttocks kneaded, your legs stretched, your shoulders and neck released, your hands massaged, your face touched, and your back smoothed out, your range of pleasure enlarges. The awakening of each area enables you to experience greater pleasure in other parts of your body and naturally enhances and deepens lovemaking.

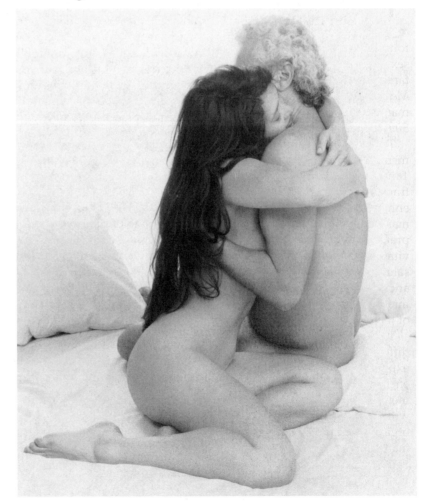

Chapter 2

BEYOND THE MIGHTY ORGASM:
AN ORIENTAL LOOK AT SEX

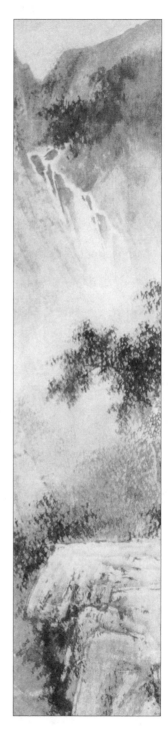

For thousands of years, the Chinese have practiced erotic techniques that enhance sexuality and overall well-being. The legendary Yellow Emperor, who lived more than four thousand years ago, was personally interested in ways to use sex to maintain radiant health. His wisest health ministers created the famous teachings known as *The Yellow Emperor's Classic of Internal Medicine.* His advisers on sexual activities compiled the ancient Taoist manuals known as *The Classic of the Plain Girl* and *The Counsels of a Simple Girl.*

The Classic of the Plain Girl inspired a great deal of sexual experimentation and led to various Taoist and Hindu practices known as Tantra. Tantra means weaving—the weaving of two people who transform sex into a lovemaking sacrament. Tantric erotic practices enhance sexual intimacy through sexual positions, scents, images, massage techniques, stories, visualizations, and other ways. Tantric practices treat sexuality as an art form, an aesthetic intimacy and vitality that celebrates love. Eastern sexuality is playful, intimate, and sacred, inviting couples to touch, smell, and move together. The ancient Tantric art of lovemaking encourages playful sounds and interactions, creating not only intimacy but harmony with the spirit of the heart.

The traditional Eastern and Western views of sexuality are quite different. After intercourse, for instance, a Taoist Chinese man may express gratitude for having "received the nectar of the woman's enchanted garden." While Western sexuality focuses on the attainment of orgasm as a goal, traditional Chinese sexology is concerned with the quality of the process of unfolding and opening up. It views orgasm not as an end in itself but as a sacred interplay of opposites: man and woman, hard and soft, giving and receiving.

In the West, sex is often looked at as a game with set roles and positions. Men and women frequently use strategies, intrigue, and

In their search into the art of lovemaking, the ancient Chinese Taoists went beyond foods and herbs, even beyond erotic techniques . . . by consciously maneuvering the human body's chi, or life-energy. They did this to enhance sexual arousal, control orgasm and intensify ecstasy for both men and women.

—Valentin Chu
The Yin-Yang Butterfly

seduction to obtain sex. With such a mind-set, the act of making love often creates conflicts between the emotions and the body. "Sex as a goal-oriented performance is the usual substitute when sex with emotional commitment either fails to develop or is deliberately avoided," noted William Masters and Virginia Johnson in *The Pleasure Bond.* Preconceived expectations—all the props, all the things you should have, should say, should do—create barriers and frustrations.

Most Western-influenced cultures do not accept sexuality as a healthy and self-expressive part of life. Western sexuality often involves unconscious scripts, the abuse of substances like alcohol that numb the body and mind, and misguided beliefs that sex is sinful or dirty. Boys learn negative egocentric attitudes about sex and develop mental strategies of performance, conquest, and control. Girls learn to distrust their sexuality, are taught that sex is immoral or uncontrollable, or view sex as a way to control their mate.

Western men are often preoccupied with their external affairs and thus are not in touch with their feelings or bodies. Sexual and emotional intimacy are unfamiliar to them. Since men tend to be sexually linear and goal-oriented, traditional Chinese sexology focuses especially on giving men advice and guidance. A man's sexual vulnerability is partly due to having genitals that are outside his body, not contained within. He cannot hide his erection, nor can he fake it.

According to ancient Taoist sexology, one of the fundamental sexual differences between men and women is how they reach orgasm. A man's sexual fluids are released out of his body, whereas a woman's fluids are recirculated within her reproductive system. After an orgasm, a man may feel drained and exhausted, ready to fall asleep. Women, on the other hand, are often rejuvenated and revitalized after an orgasm. A woman can masturbate frequently without damaging her body. From the Eastern point of view, when a man ejaculates excessively, he drains his energy and eventually ages and weakens his body, particularly his immune system.

Fortunately, acupressure points and dietary adjustments can strengthen a man's reproductive and immune systems. By conserving semen and consciously ejaculating less, a man trades a few seconds of intense pleasure for many comprehensive benefits. Preserving semen actually strengthens a man's body, enabling him to live a healthier, longer life and develop greater vitality, alertness, and mental clarity.

The more a man gives his partner acupressure and has intercourse without ejaculating, the more attentive, intimate, and loving he becomes. Both acupressure and intercourse are tremendously powerful ways of giving pleasure and healing energy. If a man can deeply fulfill his partner without dispersing his own reserves (containing sperm and testosterone), his hormones will continue to drive him affectionately to his mate.

According to ancient Chinese sexology, a man and a woman must spend time playing together, being sensual and loving, before engaging in intercourse. Loveplay or foreplay is fundamental to intimacy, enabling couples to greet, touch, exchange vital energy, and thereby attune themselves to each other.

The Classic of the Plain Girl compares male and female sexual energies to fire and water, two polar elements in nature. A woman's erotic energy is like water, it says. Just as it takes time for water to be heated, it takes time for a woman to become fully aroused. Once water is heated, however, it retains its warmth. A woman's sexual pleasure is like a vast deep ocean, and she savors it much longer than a man does his. A man's pleasure burns hot and fast. Left to his own designs, he tends to climax much faster than his partner. After ejaculating, his sexual energy cools quickly, often leaving him depleted and drained.

Chinese erotic lovemaking goes beyond genital stimulation to provide powerful expressions of affection. It can awaken transformative spiritual experiences while serving as an excellent physical workout and full-body massage. The ancient art of lovemaking uses inner awareness, deep breathing, meditation, massage, and body positions to stimulate certain acupressure points for obtaining radiant physical health and spiritual union with one's partner.

Lovers who learn to provide complete and mutual sexual ecstasy may also gain intimations of divine experience.

—Daniel P. Reid
The Tao of Health, Sex, and Longevity

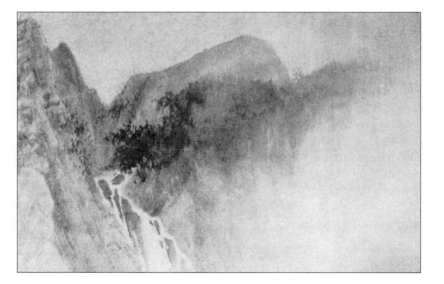

DELIGHT IN THE JOURNEY:
LETTING GO OF GOAL-ORIENTED SEXUALITY

Intimacy with another—the closeness of living the shared moments, each as it arises, the easy comfort of being known without the disguises of attempted 'perfection,' the willingness to be where I am without a blueprint or an image to be fulfilled—this particular joy is what is so new in my life.

—Elizabeth K. Blugental
On Intimacy and Death

The *Acupressure for Lovers* approach to sexuality focuses on enhancing intimacy. I believe that goal-oriented sex and intimacy are mutually exclusive. Expectations and destinations are future-oriented; they take you away from the present moment that you share with your partner.

"Delighting in the journey" means being mindful of every moment with your loved one. Open yourselves to each other, with neither expectations nor an agenda except to be present in each other's company. Enjoy the feel of your love in each touch, caress, and embrace. Breathe deeply into each sensation of pleasure, and allow each touch to represent and embody the warmth and closeness of your bond. Allow orgasm to become only one part of the experience, not the goal. Release is part of the pleasure of sex and intimacy, but by allowing yourself to focus on the pleasure before and after orgasm—by relaxing your exclusive focus on the orgasm—you will intensify the orgasm in addition to all other sensual facets of the experience.

If the joys of sex are not rooted in the heart but are used solely for momentary physical release and pleasure, relationships are limited and self-referential; they eventually become superficial, hollow, and temporary. But when sexual interaction is a sacred exchange and partners regularly set aside special time and energy to engage fully with each other, they can move toward a shared experience of deep intimacy.

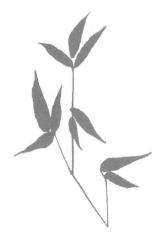

Chapter 3

STIMULATING YOUR SEXUAL ENERGY

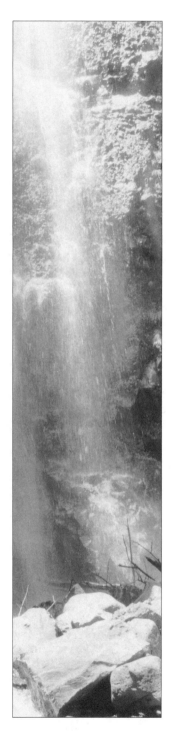

*T*his chapter is for those who want to use acupressure by themselves to increase their sexual vitality and aliveness. They may be separated from their partner or between partners, or their partner is not interested in practicing acupressure. They may simply be more committed to self-care and personal growth than their partner. If your partner is open to acupressure, however, both of you can practice the exercises in this chapter.

EMOTIONAL INTIMACY

The more ways partners express their innermost selves to each other, the deeper their intimacy can grow. For an intimate relationship to be stable, however, both partners must first know, honor, and nurture themselves. Sadly, our culture teaches people to ignore their feelings, to deny their anger, affection, and hurt. So many people are out of touch with their feelings and find it awkward to express them to others. If you cannot experience your own feelings and be aware of them yourself, how can you share them with your partner? An awareness of your own feelings is absolutely necessary for emotional intimacy.

Deep breathing can open you to your innermost feelings. Close your eyes, and focus your attention on your chest or belly. As you breathe deeply into your heart, imagine your breath reaching your feelings, massaging them, loosening them. Continue breathing slowly and deeply into these areas and feelings. Describe to yourself the sensations that develop inside your chest and belly.

The power of touch can also cultivate body awareness. By holding acupressure points on yourself as well as on your partner, you can anchor your feelings, open yourself to a greater awareness of sensations, and balance your emotions.

Since the heart governs the emotions, the acupressure points for emotional healing are located at the level of the heart, in the chest and upper back between the shoulder blades. In people who have been emotionally hurt, abused, or traumatized, these points often feel like knots. You can open withheld feelings and release tensions in this area by practicing the following exercises once or twice a day.

Reawakening Emotional Sensitivity

1. Place two tennis balls one inch apart on a thick towel. Put a folded sock between the balls to separate them, and roll the tennis balls up in the towel like a tight burrito. Alternatively, you can cover and twist the balls together in another sock.

2. Gently lie down on the tennis balls, centering them between your shoulder blades and spine. With your knees bent and your eyes closed, practice long deep breathing as you very slowly roll yourself up and down over the balls.

3. For 2 or 3 minutes, rock over the balls along the length of your back. Concentrate the pressure on your upper back between your shoulder blades. Keep your eyes closed, and breathe deeply.

4. Immediately after you remove the balls, cover yourself with a sheet or a blanket and relax for 5 to 10 minutes, as if you were going to take a nap.

When you fear that your ability to love or to be loved is threatened, when you fear, for example, expressing your own love or receiving love from another, you experience physical discomfort or pain in the region of your chest, near your heart.

—Gary Zukav
Seat of the Soul

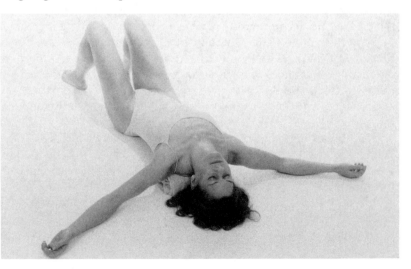

DAILY STRETCHES

Without regular stretching, our bodies become stiff and tense and tire easily. These yoga stretches prepare your body to be more relaxed and open to intimacy. Regular daily stretching awakens your body's circulation in new ways and contributes to fuller, richer lovemaking experiences.

As you stretch, close your eyes and focus on the feelings in your body. Don't force your body into stretching positions and don't strain it. Let it stretch as far as it wants to, while you accept its limitations. Stretch slowly and moderately, so that you feel some small degree of stretch but not enough to be painful. If you experience pain, you are pushing too hard. Be gentle, so that the stretches are comfortable.

These stretching exercises should not be practiced on a full stomach. Allow at least an hour after eating before you do them—two, if you have eaten a big meal with a lot of heavy food. Nor should you stuff yourself immediately after doing these exercises. Gentle stretching releases a great deal of healing energy. Eating a lot of heavy food immediately afterward often blocks this energy in the stomach, causing nausea. Thus, after practicing these exercises, wait at least an hour before eating a substantial meal. If you get hungry before then, have some soup, tea, or a piece of fruit.

These gentle exercises are quite safe when you follow the common sense guidelines. Contraindications to specific stretches will be clearly noted. If you have any concern about practicing these stretches or suffer a medical condition, be sure to consult your doctor.

When you feel tightness or resistance, focus on your breath and breathe deeply. Imagine you are breathing into and out of the tightness. Long deep breathing is key to releasing tightness in nerves and muscles.

If you feel lightheaded after stretching or if you feel new tingling sensations moving through your body, immediately lie down on your back, cover yourself, close your eyes, and let yourself relax. A short nap or even 10 minutes of repose will allow healing energy to flow and balance. Dizziness or lightheadedness can result when the energy bound up inside a point is released and then circulates throughout your body. The circulation of this vital energy can refresh your whole body, clear your mind, and make you feel new again.

The ancient Taoists believed that every part of the body, including the sex organs, could be strengthened and improved by correct exercise.

—Jolan Chang
The Tao of Love and Sex

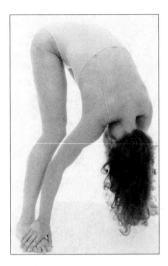

Standing Spread Squats

1. Stand with your feet spread one yard apart.

2. Slowly bend at the hips, bringing your hands to your feet, right hand on the right foot, left hand on your left foot. (Caution: If you have a history of lower back problems, bend your knees before you lean over. Once you are down, slowly straighten your legs to get a gentle stretch. Be sure to bend your knees again before you come up, to prevent lower back strain.)

3. Squat several times in this position, with your head hanging down, exhaling as you go down, inhaling as you come up.

Benefits: These squats stretch the inner thigh muscles, and open the spleen, liver, and kidney meridians, all essential channels for cultivating sexual vitality.

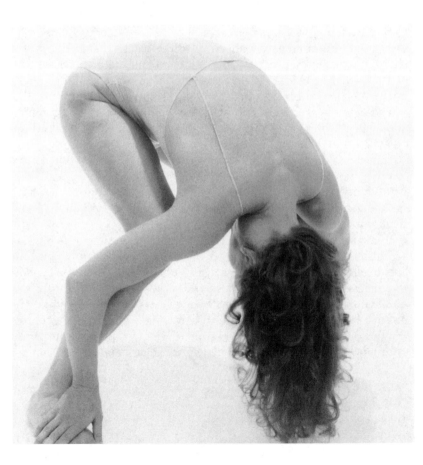

Butterfly Pose

1. Sit on the floor with your knees bent, and bring the bottoms of your feet together. Keep the sides of your feet on the floor and your knees as close to the floor as possible. Pull your feet in toward your genitals.

2. Hold the point (Sp 4) on the arches of your feet with your thumbs. Use your fingers to press the point between the fourth and fifth metatarsal bones on the tops of your feet (GB 41).

3. Inhale and straighten your spine, bringing the chest up and out.

4. Exhale as you bend forward, dropping your head forward toward your big toes.

5. Continue to breathe slowly and deeply with this movement for one minute. Then sit straight in this posture and breathe deeply.

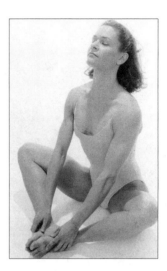

Benefits: This exercise stretches the "sex nerve" in the inner thigh as well as the kidney, liver, and spleen meridians. Stretching these channels directly benefits the sexual reproductive system for both men and women.

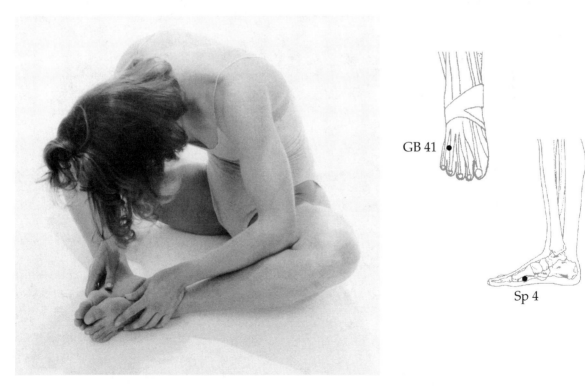

GB 41

Sp 4

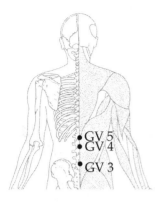

GV 5
GV 4
GV 3

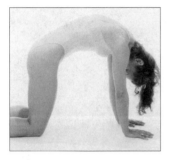

Cat-Cow

This exercise stimulates the Gates of Life points (GV 3–GV 5) along the spine. Cat-Cow also strengthens the reproductive system, the lower back, and the abdominal area.

1. Place yourself on the floor on your hands and knees. Position your hands directly below your shoulders and your knees beneath your hips.
2. Inhale as you arch your back toward the floor and raise your head up.
3. Exhale as you let your head drop down and round your back toward the ceiling.
4. Establish a smooth rhythm of inhaling as your head comes up, and exhaling as your head goes down. Continue the exercise for about one minute.

Benefits: This spinal exercise particularly benefits the female reproductive system. Practicing it can give a pleasurable, freeing feeling in the abdominal and vaginal regions.

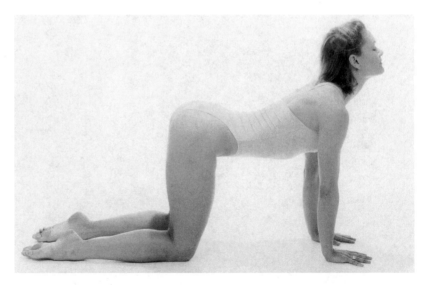

Locust Pose

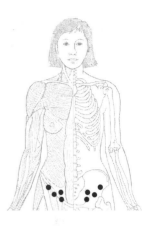

The following posture powerfully presses a series of acupressure points in the groin and pubic area. Such pressure is effective for increasing the energy flow into your genitals. Avoid doing this exercise if you find that it strains your back or aggravates any existing back pain.

1. Lie on your stomach with your feet together. Rest your head on either your chin or your forehead, whichever is more comfortable.

2. Ball your hands into fists, and put them under your hips so that they fit inside the front hip bones near the groin.

3. As you inhale deeply, lift your straightened legs as high as possible, keeping your legs straight and feet together. (Caution: Raise one leg at a time if you have had back problems.)

4. Keep your legs up and breathe deeply into your hara (lower abdomen) for about 30 seconds.

5. Inhale deeply, and raise your legs up further.

6. Let your legs return to the floor. Immediately turn your head to the side and place your hands by your sides. Completely relax for at least 3 minutes. Let yourself go as you deeply relax.

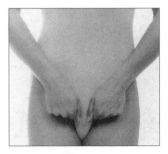

Benefits: This exercise helps relieve genital or abdominal discomfort, sexual frustration, groin pain, and low sexual desire.

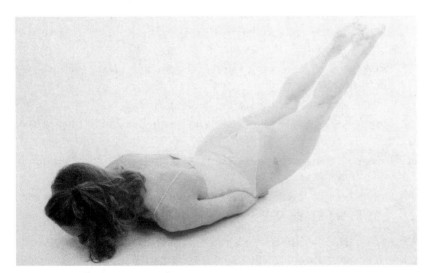

Bow Pose

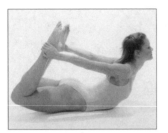

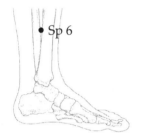

• Sp 6

Do the Butterfly and Cat-Cow exercises to prepare your body for this powerful posture. (Caution: Do not practice this exercise if you are over two months pregnant or have a history of back problems.)

1. Lie on the floor on your stomach, with your forehead on the ground. Bend your knees, and bring your feet toward your buttocks.

2. Inhale, and grab hold of the tops of your feet from the sides. Bring your fingers over the shins to hold Sp 6.

3. Arch yourself back like a bow. Begin rocking, inhaling as you rock back and exhaling as you rock forward. Breathe through your nose. Continue rocking for 15 seconds.

4. Release the pose slowly. Immediately lie down comfortably on your stomach with your head turned to the side. Relax for at least 3 minutes with your hands by your sides, palms facing up. Consciously breathe through your nose into and out of the lower abdomen, during this deep relaxation period.

Benefits: This posture strengthens the spine and reproductive system as well as benefits the circulation and nervous system.

Sex Nerve Stroke and Stretch

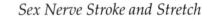

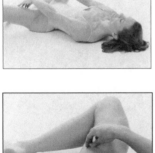

1. Lie on the floor on your back. Bend your knees, placing the soles of your feet together.

2. Relax your legs, keeping the feet together but letting your knees fall to the sides.

3. Place your hands on the insides of your knees.

4. Inhale as you lightly stroke your inner thighs slowly toward your genitals.

5. Exhale as you return your hands to your knees without touching your thighs.

6. Continue stroking up the inside of your thighs with your eyes closed for a couple of minutes.

Benefits: This self-massage stretches the sex nerve and traces the pathways of the kidney, spleen, and liver meridians. The pleasurable exercise can enable both men and women to cultivate greater sexual ease with their partner.

Bridge Pose

1. Lie on your back with your knees bent so that the soles of your feet are flat on the floor.

2. Bring your arms above your head on the floor. Relax your arms with your elbows bent and your palms facing up.

3. Inhale as you arch your pelvis up, bringing your back off the floor. Hold for several seconds.

4. Exhale as you slowly come down. Continue to inhale up and exhale down for 1 minute.

5. Let yourself completely relax on your back with your eyes closed for a few minutes.

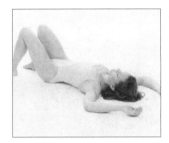

Benefits: This exercise relieves fatigue, nervous exhaustion, irritability, shoulder pain or ache, excessive anger, hypertension, pelvic tension, and impotence. It is also good for someone with low sexual desire, cold hands, or cold feet. This exercise increases resistance to colds and flu.

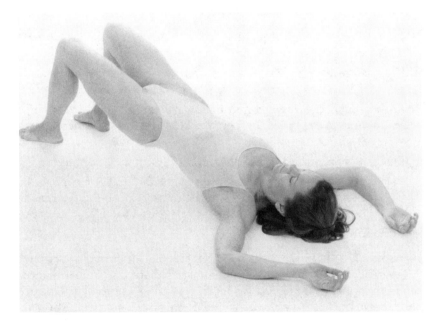

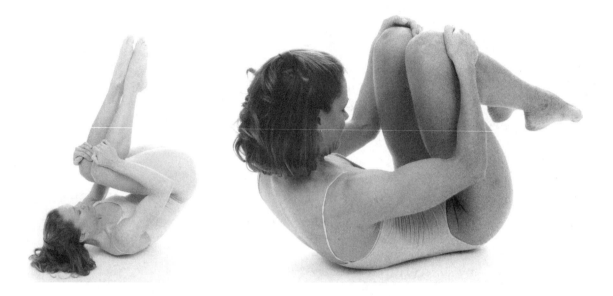

Rock and Roll

1. Lie on your back on a padded surface. Bend your knees so that your feet are flat on the floor.

2. Use your arms to pull your knees up to your chest. Lift your head up off the floor to round your back, and rock on your spine.

3. Rock your body forward and backward for 1 minute, applying stimulation to the points on your back. If you have a tight spot on your back, rock back onto it.

4. Relax in the posture and breathe long and deep for 1 minute.

5. Release the posture, and relax completely. Lie on your back with your head on the floor, your knees bent, feet flat on the floor, and eyes closed for a few minutes. Feel your blood and energy circulate.

Benefits: This exercise massages the internal organs, presses the points along the spine, stretches the muscles there, and helps balance the thyroid gland. It is good for relieving stiffness in the back, neck, shoulders, and legs. The increased flexibility and circulation it produces can certainly benefit your love life.

RESTORING THE BODY'S NATURAL RESPONSIVENESS

Sit comfortably on a chair during the first three steps of this self-acupressure routine.

1. Rub B 47 and B 23. Using the backs of your hands, rub your lower back points briskly up and down for 1 minute, creating heat from the friction. Next, using your thumbs or your fingers, firmly press on the outer edge of the large vertical muscles along the spine in the lower back to stimulate these points. Press on both sides for at least 1 minute.

2. Briskly rub St 36. Bring your left leg straight out in front of you, resting the heel on the floor. Place your right heel on the left St 36 point, outside your leg below your knee. With your heel, briskly rub this point for 1 minute. Then switch sides, and do the same on your right leg with your left heel.

3. Press K 3 with K 1. Comfortably position your left foot on your right thigh. Then place your left thumb on K 3, between the Achilles tendon and the inside anklebone, angling your pressure into the area underneath the inside anklebone. Use your right thumb to press K 1 in the center of the sole of the foot. Hold these points firmly for 1 minute as you concentrate on breathing deeply. Then switch to hold K 3 with K 1 on your left foot for 1 minute. These reflexology and acupressure points cultivate sexual energy especially when the lower back points are stimulated as well.

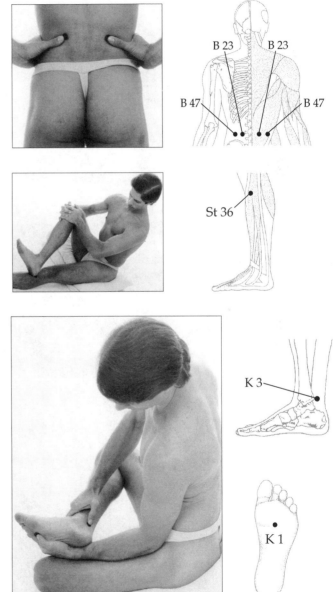

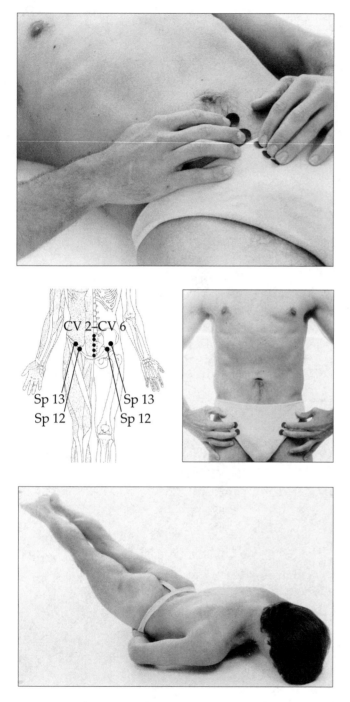

CV 2–CV 6

Sp 13
Sp 12

Sp 13
Sp 12

4. Press CV 2–CV 6. Lie down comfortably on your back with your knees bent, feet flat on the floor. Place the fingertips of one hand just above the center of your pubic bone on CV 2, CV 3, and CV 4, and the fingers of your other hand just above that, between your belly button and pubic bone, on CV 5 and CV 6. Close your eyes, and breathe deeply as you apply firm pressure on these Sea of Intimacy points for 1 to 2 minutes.

Applying heat to these lower abdominal points fortifies the sexual-reproductive system. Try using a hot compress, a hot water bottle, a heating pad, or a hand-held hair dryer to warm these potent points gently and carefully for a few minutes, as you consciously breathe deeply.

5. Hold Sp 12 and Sp 13. With all of your fingertips, press directly on the thick ropy ligament located in the groin at the center of the leg crease at the top of your thigh. Hold for 1 minute. While pressing these points you'll feel a strong pulsation from the large artery that runs between these points and your genitals.

To stimulate these groin points more deeply, lie flat on your abdomen and place your fists in your groin. Bring your forehead or your chin to the floor and your feet together. Then inhale and raise your feet up with your thighs off the ground. This will put pressure on these potency points. Breathe long and deep, with your legs up, for 30 seconds. Then let your legs down and relax your hands at your sides. Adjust your body comfortably, and completely relax for 2 minutes.

6. Press points B 27–B 34. Lie on your back with your knees bent, feet flat on the floor. Lift your pelvis up, and place your hands—one on top of the other, palms down, fingers of one hand crossed on top of the fingers of the other—under the sacrum, at the base of your spine. Slowly lower your pelvis onto your hands. Then let your knees sway from side to side for 1 minute as you breathe deeply into your belly. A variation (with your hands still under the base of the spine) is to bring your feet several inches off the ground and rotate your knees in a large slow circular motion.

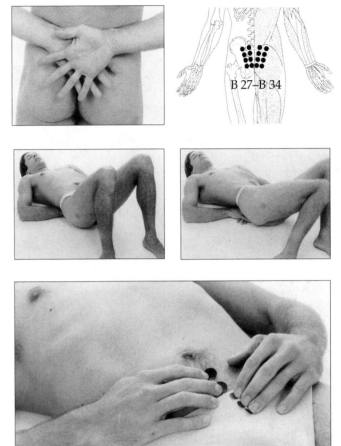

B 27–B 34

7. Repeat Step 4. Gradually press CV 2–CV 6 firmly once again for 1 minute. Breathe deeply into your lower belly while you hold these Sea of Intimacy points to achieve greater sexual responsiveness and pleasure.

Body awareness and sexual energy are the foundation for a vital love life. Continue to practice the exercises in this chapter as you age to maintain your sexual vitality.

Chapter 4

BUILDING INTIMACY

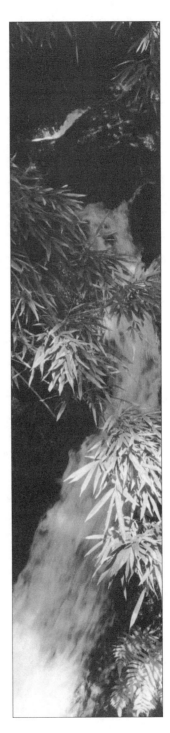

*A*cupressure opens many spiritual experiences in our sexuality," Judy says. "When our bodies are totally relaxed together after practicing acupressure on each other, a powerful healing energy circulates through us, creating an ecstatic experience. Every time I give Richard acupressure, our sexual movements seem limitless. Our bodies flow with each other, and Richard touches me so much more sensually. Something changes within him."

Richard confirms this view. "I get an afterglow feeling from acupressure that really slows me down and enables me to enjoy Judy's body. Just as meditating before a meal lets me concentrate on every detail of the food, using acupressure relaxes me and lets me feel my own body and Judy's."

"The more that we experiment with holding each other's points during sex," Judy adds, "the deeper our spiritual experiences become. With acupressure, we tend to make love much longer. We are more intimate, and we are both sexually happier. Our bodies seem to merge without effort. The more my acupressure points open, the deeper our intimacy seems to evolve, adding a strong spiritual dimension to our love relationship."

INTIMACY AND SACRED SEXUALITY

Because it is based on mutual caring, acupressure generates deep feelings of affection and love. Learn where your partner tends to collect tension, which are the best points to relieve it, and exactly how he or she prefers to be touched. Knowing this, you can help your partner more effectively. The better feedback you give each other the more new pleasurable areas you will discover. The more you give and receive, the more your experience will build understanding and confidence, and the better your lives together will be physically, emotionally, and sexually.

Acupressure's touch conveys security, compassion, attentiveness, healing, and deep relaxation. Because the touch is applied gradually and is pointed in toward the center of the body, it creates a feeling of acceptance, enabling you and your partner to open up and communicate with each other.

Touch that is connected to the heart communicates love and unconditional acceptance. It can transmit the deepest, most tender part of your inner being, attuning you and your partner to each other spiritually. Acupressure can dissolve performance anxieties, provide greater body contact, and open the flow of the life force—the key for energetically uniting a couple. Acupressure also expands your body's awareness through increased circulation, heightening your ability to be intimate, sensual, and erotic—all without drugs. Acupressure is a physical way to channel and anchor your love.

IMPROVING SEXUAL COMMUNICATION

By providing physical support that is safe and nurturing, acupressure can enable couples to talk about sex more easily and openly and to break through unproductive ways of relating to each other. Steve, a forty-two-year-old accountant, was constipated and did not feel sexual. But he wanted to respond to his wife's desire to make love, and he would try to give her pleasure and satisfy her. After more than an hour of caressing and stimulating Jane, he managed to get a slight erection, enough to go inside of her. When he entered her, Jane became highly aroused. Steve then assumed she had had an orgasm, his semi-erection left him, and his penis slipped out. Despite his physical inability, he felt close to his wife physically and emotionally and told her so. Unfortunately, she did not respond in the same way. "I can't believe you're saying that. I'm feeling so frustrated!" she said.

Steve might have become defensive or sarcastic, or he might have turned away and felt wounded and attacked. Instead, Steve reached out to hold Jane's hand. The physical contact enabled them to feel connected as they talked. He told her, "I'm terribly upset. After trying so hard to satisfy and please you, we're both frustrated and agitated. I was loving you with all my heart. I did everything I could to turn you on."

"That's just it," Jane replied. "You were so focused on stimulating me, on pleasing me, trying to do all the right things—I never felt you

The practice of intimacy is a mind-fulness exercise in which your purpose is to be open and honest with your partner and to pay scrupulous attention to him or her. Willfully appreciate this person, whether you are together or not. Appreciation is a doorway into the heart.

—Frank Andrews, Ph.D.
The Art and Practice of Loving

were really here. I think it scares me," she confessed, "when you seem in another world, not really in touch with me. I'm not just a body that you play with, stimulate, and arouse." She squeezed his hand lovingly. "It all felt great, Steve. I just wish you would slow down, look into my eyes, and be with me. Techniques for arousing me are not what I need from you. It's the intimacy, the closeness, that turns me on.

"While you were playing with me, I was wondering why you weren't getting hard," she continued. "I found myself caught between enjoying your touch and worrying what was going on with you. You were trying so persistently to make me come, yet I wasn't able to let go."

"I just realized that the times you come unexpectedly are when we are relating heart to heart," Steve said. "I think my intestines being a wreck block my sexual energy."

"Would you like me to hold some acupressure points on your belly to relieve your stomachache?" she offered.

Jane and Steve's sex life and health have been improved by using acupressure. They often start making love by sitting close together, holding each other's points while they talk. Acupressure's healing contact heightens their sensual awareness and pleasure.

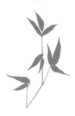

MAKING EYE CONTACT

The eyes, as William Blake put it, "are dim windows of the soul." When you gaze into his or her eyes, you can see your loved one's inner world and tune in to what your partner is feeling. Avoiding each other's eyes reflects an unspoken distrust, a barrier between you.

Eye gazing brings you into the present moment. It enables you to perceive your partner's moods, expectations, and intentions. When you look into your partner's eyes, notice whether they shift nervously or are cast downward with reservation, whether they well up with tears of emotion or are attentive. Maintaining close loving contact while eye gazing can bring about an extraordinary connection in your partnership.

Conscious lovers should try to maintain contact with each other in as many ways as possible during their lovemaking, and the eyes are perhaps the most important way of doing so; in tantric loving, the eyes are considered a primary organ of intimacy.

—Charles and Caroline Muir
Tantra: The Art of Conscious Loving

Maintaining eye contact while breathing deeply and touching or talking is an essential step for creating a more intimate bond. Try the following breathing exercise to cultivate a calm, loving spirit:

1. Sit close together on thick pillows, either on top of your bed or on a carpeted floor.

2. Face each other with your spines straight. Place the palms of your own hands together at the center of your chest. The backs of your thumbs press firmly against your breastbone, holding CV 17, at the level of your heart.

3. Gaze into your partner's eyes.

4. Concentrate on breathing slow, even, deep breaths into your heart for about 3 minutes. Make each breath longer and deeper than the last one. With each deep breath, feel yourself becoming clearer as you gaze into your partner's eyes. Remember, you are breathing in life itself.

5. After a few minutes, let your hands drift down gracefully toward your partner's lap until you are holding each other's hands. Continue to breathe deeply together, and hold hands as you gaze into each other's eyes for a couple of minutes. Then take as much time as you want to touch each other's faces, hands, arms, chests, and shoulders while breathing deeply and maintaining eye contact.

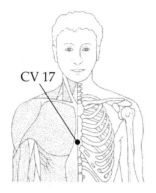

CV 17

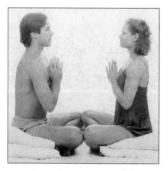

The eye of love makes every person in the world friendly and attractive.

—Sai Baba

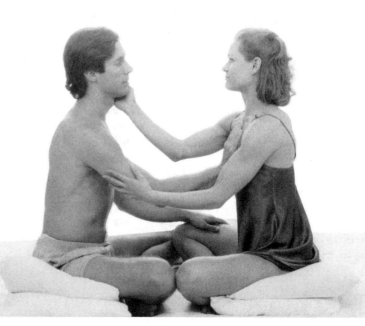

HEALING SOUNDS

Sound vibrations generated from the vocal cords can open the spiritual centers called chakras, awakening a symphony of spiritual energy in your body.

When you and your partner make sounds while embracing and breathing deeply together, extraordinary communication can occur. Through your sounds you can intimately express your innermost self, and the sound vibrations you release enable your partner to feel your body. By opening the body's life force, these vibrations often create powerful, transformative experiences for couples.

In a private space where you can both feel free to make sounds, cuddle close in any comfortable position, maximizing your body contact. Hold any two acupressure points on your partner while you make harmonious sounds together. Close your eyes, and begin long deep breathing, inhaling and exhaling together in sync for a minute. After you inhale deeply, make a long releasing "ahhh" sound on the exhale, letting go of internalized stress. Keep your eyes closed. As you and your partner make this sound together, increase the volume and enjoy its harmonious healing vibrations. Try making other sounds together, and experience their healing effects.

Experiment with making sounds while you are massaging, meditating, or making love. You may find that you enjoy the effects of different sounds for different activities. For instance, "ahhh" releases stress and opens you to deeper pleasure. Sighing "ohhh" while making love also enables you to take in more pleasure. The sound "youuu" opens you to accept pleasure from your partner in a very intimate, powerful, erotic way. When you make the "ummm" sound, you savor the pleasure you are receiving. Try these healing sounds in any of the love positions in this book to heighten your pleasure and spiritual experience.

When we give expression to the voice within, it emerges from the place deep inside that is at One with the Great Mystery, with God, with All and everything. . . . The human voice is one of our finest tools for healing the body and spirit.

—Joy Gardner-Gordon
The Healing Voice

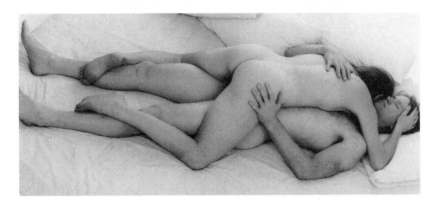

IMAGERY, MOVEMENT, AND MEDITATION

Moving your body enables your vital life force to flow, increasing both your circulation and your capacity to open yourself to your partner. In the following visualization, your breath and body make conscious contact. You may want to tape-record it so that you can both follow it unencumbered by the book.

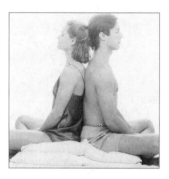

Begin by stretching your bodies for several minutes. Either create your own movements, or do the stretches at the end of this chapter. Now sit up comfortably, back to back, with your spines together, maximizing your contact and support. Close your eyes and practice the following visualization:

Begin long deep breathing together. . . . As you breathe the life force into your bodies, be conscious of your spinal column. . . . With your hands resting in your lap, palms facing up, continue to breathe as slowly and as deeply as possible. Let your breath open your body's awareness.

Breathe into the base of your spine. Breathe as deeply as you want your relationship to be guided, gifted, and graced. As you imagine your breath going into the base of your spine, feel your legs and feet. . . . Now breathe slowly into the depths of your belly, letting the energy of the breath spill into your genitals. Feel your sexual vitality flow through you and your partner.

Visualization is the heart of the bio-computer. The human brain programs and self-programs through its images. Visualization is the ultimate consciousness tool.

—Michael Samuels, M.D., and Nancy Samuels
Seeing with the Mind's Eye

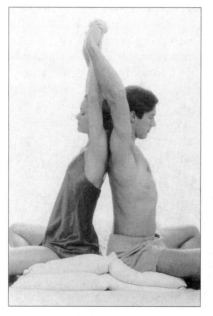

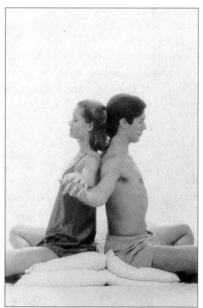

Now, inhale as you stretch your arms up to the sky and reach back, connecting with your partner's hands. Exhale as your hands float back down into your lap. Once again, inhale as your hands stretch up and grasp hold of your partner's hands. Exhale as your hands float back down into your lap, relaxing your shoulders and letting the energy in your body circulate.

With each inhalation, breathe love into your heart. . . . Let that energy circulate into your partner as you exhale. Send this energy into your partner's upper back, imagining your love flowing into your partner's heart.

Inhale again, leaning your head back and gently making contact with your partner's head. Let the energy inside your head go as you exhale and relax. Once again inhale deeply as you roll your eyes back, gently stretching your eye muscles. Exhale as you slowly let both your heads fall forward. Slowly bring your hands in back of you, holding hands comfortably with your partner. Continue to breathe deeply as you communicate love for your partner through your touch.

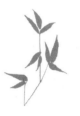

SPIRITUAL POINTS

Using acupressure in your lovemaking can give your spiritual relationship a boost and enables you to tap into life's infinite supply of universal healing energy. When your bodies open to this universal healing energy, sex can become a mystical experience, uniting your bodies and souls in oneness.

A relationship that has a spiritual center can be an emotional sanctuary for both partners, a safe haven for nurturing each other's personal growth. As you attune yourself spiritually by meditating or practicing conscious movements and breathing exercises, you cultivate a divine presence and clarity that you can share together.

The following acupressure points are important for experiencing and expressing the spiritual components of your relationship and balancing your emotions. Pressing these points creates a current of spiritual energy, bringing your mind and heart into closer communication. Focus on breathing deeply as you hold these points, and maintain eye contact to heighten your spiritual intimacy.

Union is the fusion of two divinities to create a third on earth; the binding together of two strong in their love against an adversary weak in its hating. 'Tis the casting away by two spirits of discord and their oneness with unity. The golden link in a chain whose first is a glance, whose last is the Infinite.

—Kahlil Gibran
A Tear and a Smile

GV 24.5

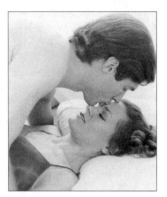

Third Eye (GV 24.5)

Location: Directly between the eyebrows, in the indentation where the bridge of the nose meets the forehead.

Benefits: Using this transformative point can enhance the spirit and morale in your love relationship. It stimulates and balances the endocrine system, especially the pituitary gland.

Applications for Spiritual Intimacy: While you are both standing or lying down, hug your partner. Place your hands behind your partner's head for support. Comfortably kiss your partner's Third Eye point, between the eyebrows. Begin with long slow kisses on the center of the forehead. Then spend a couple of minutes sucking the Third Eye point strongly. The firm suction focuses your partner's attention on this spiritually uplifting point and opens it. To heighten this experience, both of you can gently roll your eyes upward. Lift your eyebrows upward too, and breathe deeply together in sync.

You can also lightly touch the Third Eye with your middle fingertip. Encourage your partner to breathe slowly and deeply, focusing all of your attention on the point.

While making love, try holding the base of the skull while you passionately kiss the Third Eye point.

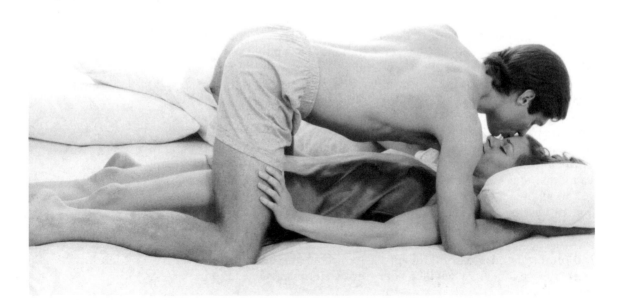

Sea of Tranquility (CV 17)

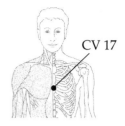

CV 17

Location: On the center of the breastbone, four finger-widths up from the base of the breastbone in an indentation.

Benefits: Holding this point can soothe and calm the spirit of the heart and increase inner joy and emotional intimacy.

Applications for Emotional Intimacy: With your fingertips, press the hollows in the center of the breastbone at the level of the heart. Adjust the amount of pressure so that it feels good to your partner. Hold this emotional balancing point for at least 2 minutes, while you synchronize breathing deeply together and gaze into each other's eyes.

A loving full-body hug is a wonderful way to stimulate the Sea of Tranquility. As you embrace, hold your partner between the shoulder blades, pressing the upper back with your fingertips.

Take off your partner's shirt. First kiss, then suck the Sea of Tranquility. After your lips stimulate the point, hug your partner chest to chest.

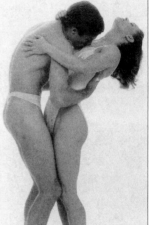

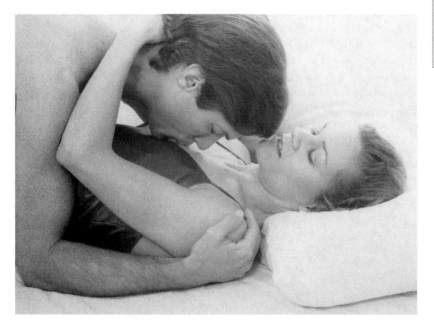

Shoulder Well (GB 21) *and Heavenly Rejuvenation* (TW 15)

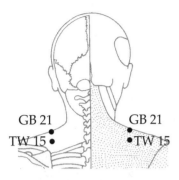

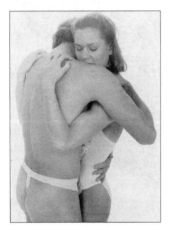

Caution: Press these points very lightly on a pregnant woman. If she is exceptionally physically fit, you can gradually apply more pressure.

Location: GB 21 is on the highest point of the top of the shoulder muscle, one inch out from the base of the lower neck. TW 15 is also on the shoulder muscle, one-half inch directly below GB 21.

Benefits: Holding these points on your partner relieves stress, uptightness, and irritability.

Applications for Spiritual Renewal:

While hugging: Whether you are standing or lying down front-to-front, hug your partner by pressing the insides of your forearms between your partner's shoulder blades. Curve your fingers, hooking your fingertips onto the tightest points above the shoulder blades. Gradually apply firm pressure as you breathe deeply together. After a couple of minutes, slowly release the pressure and hold the shoulder points lightly. End by massaging the neck and underneath the base of the skull, and then, of course, by more hugging.

While sitting: Your partner is seated in a chair. Stand behind him or her, and rest your fingertips on his or her shoulders. Use your thumbs to isolate a marble of tension in the shoulder muscles. Hold this point firmly or slowly massage it, kneading out any tension. Slowly increase the pressure, encouraging your partner to breathe deeply. End by holding the point lightly for a minute, gradually easing off.

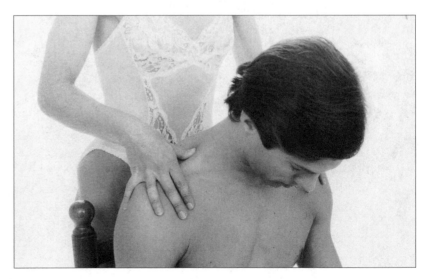

Posterior Summit (GV 19), *One Hundred Meeting* (GV 20), *Anterior Summit* (GV 21), *and Penetrating Heaven* (B 7)

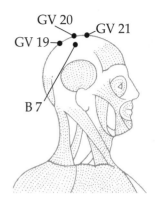

Locations: Place your left fingers behind your left ear and your right fingers behind your right ear. Move your fingertips up toward the top of the head, then feel for the hollow toward the back of the center of the top of the head. This is GV 20. GV 19 is also in a hollow, one thumb-width behind GV 20. GV 21 is one thumb-width in front of GV 20. All three points are on the midline of the skull.

Penetrating Heaven (B 7) is located on the top of the skull in a line directly upward from the back of the ears, one thumb's width outward from the center of the top of the head.

Benefits: Holding these points opens up your intuition, body wisdom, and connection with the universal flow.

Applications for Spiritual Intimacy: Spiritually oriented couples can use these points during a long embrace, during breath meditations, and during lovemaking. Since the points are gateways for transmitting spiritual energy, making sounds while holding them and long deep breathing will increase the flow of energy through them.

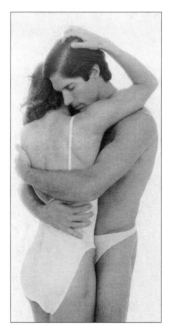

Making tones: While you are standing or lying down together, place one hand on the top of your partner's head. Close your eyes and position yourselves comfortably. Inhale deeply together. On the exhalation, make a long, sweet, open "aaah" sound in harmony with your partner. When you run out of air, inhale deeply and make the sound again. This spiritual practice deepens your breathing and creates an energetic link as the acupressure points are being held.

Hold these three points with your index, middle, and ring fingers in the hollows on the back top of your partner's head as if you were playing a flute. Use these points as you hug while either standing up or lying in bed. Holding them during lovemaking or after an orgasm opens a strong spiritual connection.

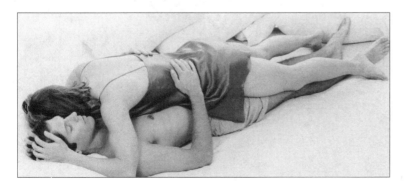

Spirit Gate (H 7)

Inner Arm

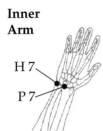

H 7

P 7

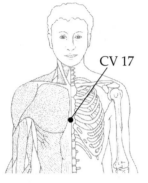

CV 17

Location: On the little-finger side of the forearm, in the dip between the wrist bone and the center of the wrist crease.

Benefits: Holding this emotional balancing point relieves fear and anxiety.

Applications for Spiritual Intimacy: With either your thumb or middle finger, grasp your partner's wrist, feeling for this powerful spiritual point on the inside of the wrist crease, near the bone that juts out directly below the pinkie. Another point to hold for increasing spiritial intimacy is located in the center of the wrist crease (P 7).

Use this tranquilizing point for coping with spiritual and emotional emergencies. When your partner is especially upset or depressed, hold it along with the Sea of Tranquility point (CV 17), on the center of the breastbone, to calm your partner.

When you are in bed with your partner, make contact with each other's feet or ankles. You can also grasp hold of your partner's wrist to stretch and stimulate the Spirit Gate points. This powerful full-body hug is a variation of Harmony Bonding: A Tantric Embrace. (See Chapter 5.)

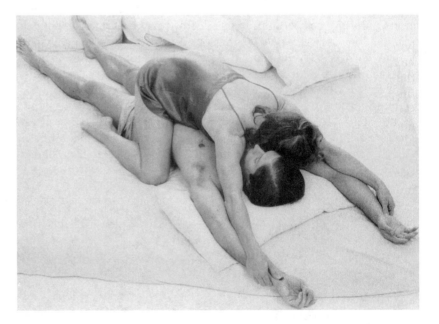

Gates of Consciousness (GB 20)

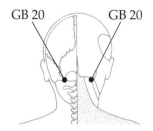

Location: Below the base of the skull, in the hollows between the two large neck muscles, 3 to 4 inches apart depending on the size of the head.

Benefits: This point is a major gate through which energy flows through the brain. While you are making love, opening the GB 20 point glorifies your experience.

Applications for Spiritual Intimacy: Have your partner sit comfortably in a chair or on a pillow on the floor. From behind your partner, place your thumbs 2 to 3 inches apart (depending upon the size of the head) underneath the base of the skull. Gently place your fingertips on your partner's temples. Slowly tilt the head backward. With your partner's eyes closed, gradually press the Gates of Consciousness in the hollow spots beneath the base of the skull. Slowly stretch the head upward, applying firm pressure to these points while you both breathe deeply in sync for 1 to 2 minutes. Then slowly bring your partner's head forward and down, to gently stretch the neck. After a minute of lightly massaging your partner's skull and temples in this position, hold the back of your partner's head in the palm of your hand. Kiss the Third Eye point (GB 24.5), between the eyebrows, for another minute.

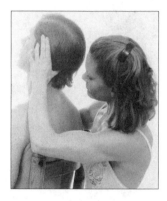

You can also hold the Gates of Consciousness while your partner is lying on his or her back. Sit at the top of the head, and gently pull the hair out from underneath the neck. Knead the muscles sensitively at the back of the neck in superslow motion, using your thumb and fingers to squeeze out any tension. Place your fingertips beneath the skull with your fingers curved, gradually pulling outward, giving the neck gentle traction. Breathe deeply in sync with your partner, holding the points until you feel the pulses on both sides synchronize and balance. After a few minutes, slowly rake your partner's skull several times, gliding your fingertips up to the top of the head, to communicate your love and support.

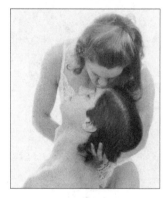

While you make love, press the Gates of Consciousness on both sides with either your thumbs or your fingertips (whatever feels more comfortable) for a few minutes. As you hold these points, encourage your partner to gently roll his or her eyes up and back, raise the eyebrows, and breathe deeply. Pressing this point enhances your five senses and heightens your consciousness, often producing a natural high.

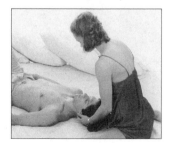

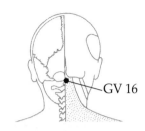

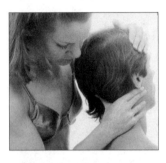

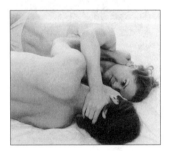

Wind Mansion (GV 16)

Location: In the center of the back of the head, in the large hollow under the base of the skull, called the medulla.

Benefits: Holding this point opens all the spiritual senses; it is good for the eyes, ears, nose, and throat.

Applications for Spiritual Intimacy:

With your partner sitting: Your partner is sitting either in a comfortable chair or on a pillow on the floor. Stand or kneel behind, and place your thumb on the hollow in the center of the back of the skull. As the palm of your other hand supports the forehead, slowly tilt your partner's head back. Gradually apply firm pressure as you rotate the head slowly in one direction and then the other.

With your partner on his or her back: Sit at your partner's head. Place the pads of your middle fingers into the large hollow in the center of the back of the skull. As you apply pressure, slowly pull the head toward you, elongating the vertebrae in the neck. Breathe long, slow, deep breaths together in sync, holding the points for 2 or 3 minutes.

While lying down in bed, facing each other: Reach around to your partner's neck. Using your middle fingers primarily, press into the large hollow in the center of the back of your partner's skull (GV 16). Once you feel your middle fingertips fit the hollow area, gradually press upward and slightly outward into the hollow spaces, giving your partner's neck traction.

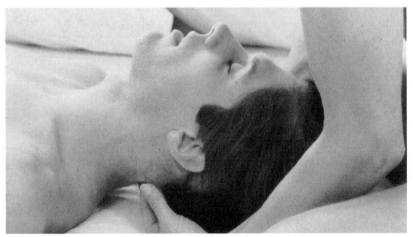

STRETCHES FOR COUPLES

These exercises for couples foster relaxation and serve as excellent preparation for lovemaking. As you practice these stretches, keep your eyes open and move more slowly than normal, being conscious of your own body. Moving slowly allows you to tune in to your partner's body and remain aware of each other's limits. By slowing down, you avoid straining each other's muscles.

These exercises are organized in a series that progresses from standing to sitting to lying down in a relaxing, intimate position. Initially, you may want to do them wearing comfortable clothing, to become accustomed to them before you do them without clothing.

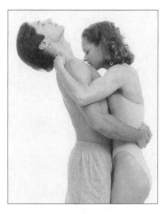

Frontal Back Arch

1. Stand close, facing each other. The taller partner spreads his or her feet apart, positioned outside the other partner's feet.

2. Place your hands on your partner's neck or shoulders with your fingers curved. Your partner's hands are placed on your lower back, giving firm support.

3. With your knees slightly bent, pelvis to pelvis, slowly arch backward, lifting your chest up and out as your partner braces backward with head forward and knees bent. Hold this position for a few seconds, as you inhale.

4. Exhale as you come back to center, stabilizing your weight.

5. Bend in the opposite direction, repeating Steps 3 and 4.

6. After a couple of minutes, switch your hand positions and repeat Steps 3 and 4 a few more times with long deep breathing.

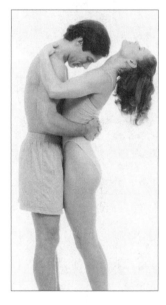

Couple's Squats

1. With your feet positioned a shoulder-width apart, distance yourself approximately one foot from your partner's toes.

2. Grasp your partner's arms above the elbows. As you hold them, slowly lean some of your weight backward, balancing with your partner, who has grasped your arms as well.

3. Slowly squat, maintaining your balance with your partner. Squat for 5 to 10 seconds, gently stretching downward.

4. Inhale deeply as you slowly come up to a comfortable standing position.

5. Repeat the squat at least one more time.

When you commit to a spiritual partnership . . . you learn the value of considering the other's position. By becoming the other person, by truly walking into the fears of the other and then returning into your own being again . . . you see each other as spiritual playmates as you work through the areas that require healing in each of you.

—Gary Zukav
Seat of the Soul

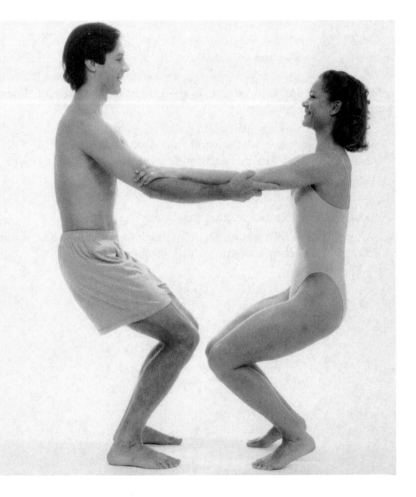

Back-to-Back Squats

1. Turn back-to-back, and interlock your arms at your elbows with your partner.
2. Lean against your partner's back, maximizing the contact and support.
3. Slowly squat, maintaining firm contact with your partner's back.
4. After 5 seconds, slowly come up, staying in balance with your partner.
5. Repeat this squat at least one more time, breathing together, with your eyes closed.

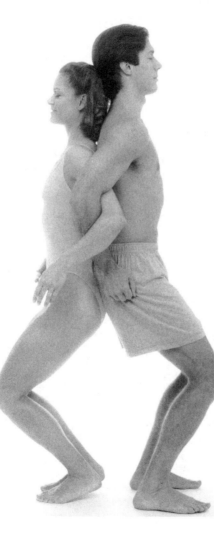

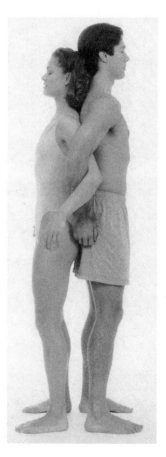

Back-to-Back Arches

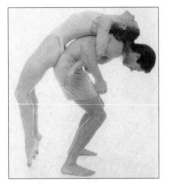

1. Again, stand back-to-back with your arms interlocked at the elbows.
2. With knees bent, one partner slowly leans forward, stretching the other partner over his or her back. Hold this position for only 3 to 5 seconds.
3. Slowly come back to center, standing upright. Take a deep breath together for stability.
4. The partner that was stretched on top now bends his or her knees and leans forward, reversing the arch.
5. Arch the back in both directions again, repeating Steps 2, 3, and 4.

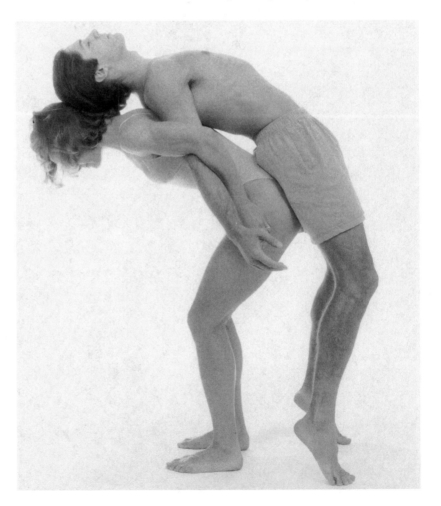

Leg Spread Pull and Stretch

1. Sit on the floor facing each other with your legs spread wide apart. The partner who is smaller or has tighter legs places the soles of his or her feet on the inner ankle area of the other partner. If both partners' legs are similar in length and flexibility, place the soles of your feet together with your legs spread wide apart.

2. Firmly grip your partner's hands. Keep your eyes open, maintaining an awareness of how your partner responds to the following stretch.

3. Take turns slowly pulling each other forward and backward. Avoid straining your partner by making the stretch as gradual as possible and staying within his or her limitations.

4. Continue pulling and stretching for about 1 minute. Then cuddle, breathe deeply together, and embrace each other to discover the wonderful benefits of these couple's stretches.

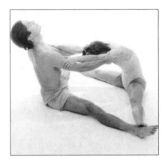

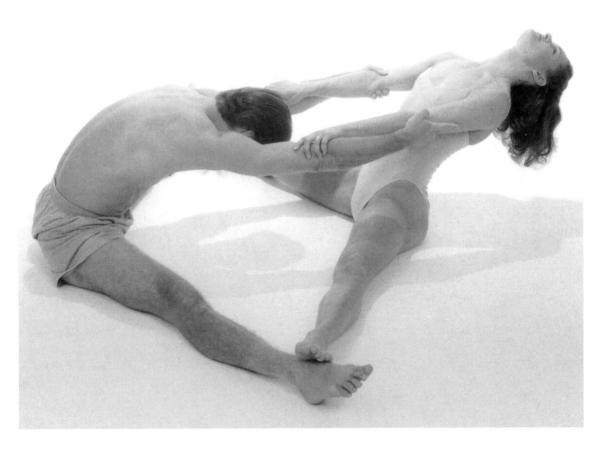

Chapter 5

PREPARING FOR LOVE

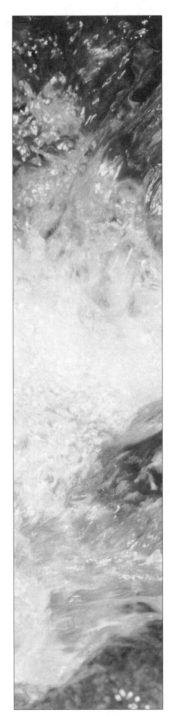

*T*his chapter is for lovers in the earliest stages of a sexual relationship as well as for those who have been together for a long time but are open to exploring new ways of interacting. In this chapter you will find an acupressure massage for releasing your partner's shoulder and neck tension, a guide to stress reduction points, a stress reduction routine, supportive couple's exercises, a spiritual attunement, and a full-body embrace called Harmony Bonding.

SHOULDER AND NECK RELEASE

Years ago, I was in love with a woman who put me through a roller-coaster ride of great highs and tremendous lows. We started each day by doing special stretching and breathing exercises together. Every morning, she would wake up negative, grumpy, and irritable. Since I adored her, on her birthday I made a commitment to give her acupressure ten nights in a row. Even though some nights I was exhausted, I managed to give her the following shoulder and neck routine. At the end of ten days, to my amazement, she was optimistic about life and cheerful in the morning, and best of all, she seemed incredibly in love with me.

Shoulder and neck tension is common for both men and women. This hands-on routine is particularly helpful for alleviating the tensions that can ruin a relationship. Try it someday when your partner comes home exhausted after work. You can also use it to relieve general stress, minor depression, aggravation, anxiety, and insomnia.

At first, this routine will take you at least a half hour to finish. But once you become familiar with the techniques (and don't have to read through all these instructions!) the eight steps will take you only 10 to 15 minutes. You can lengthen the massage, if you wish, by first

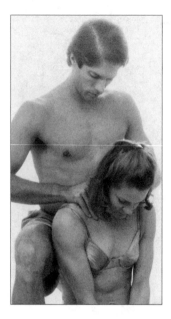

pressing some of the stress reduction points, which are listed later in this chapter.

Have your partner sit on a couple of pillows on the floor. Place the heel of your hand on top of your partner's shoulders, close to the base of the neck, with your fingertips resting on the upper chest. Gradually lean your weight inward and downward, slowly applying pressure to the top of the shoulders with the heels of your hands.

If your partner feels that he or she is getting a headache, you applied the pressure too fast or too hard. Always apply the pressure gradually, moving into and out of the points slowly.

If pressing the shoulders hurts your partner's back, take a step to the left; using the flat palm of your right hand, briskly rub the length of the back for at least a half minute to increase circulation and relieve the pain or pressure. Then gently knead the top of the shoulder muscle close to the neck in superslow motion for 1 minute.

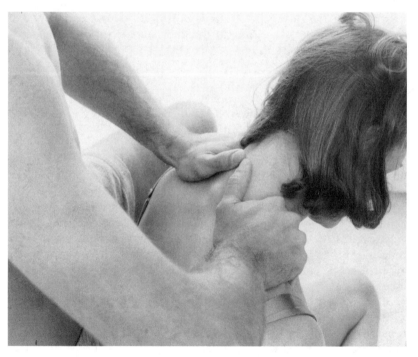

1. Upper Back Press. Take a step back from your partner. In a standing position, place both hands on top of the shoulders. Use your thumbs to press the upper back between the spine and the shoulder blades. Let your body lean into your thumbs, and gradually apply firm pressure into the large ropy muscles alongside the spine for 5 to 10 seconds at a time. Continue down the upper back, keeping your shoulders and arms relaxed.

If you or your partner feels a knot of tightness at any of these points, hold it firmly for 1 to 2 minutes as you coach him or her to take several long deep breaths.

2. Shoulder Press. Place both of your thumbs on top of your partner's shoulders, pressing into the muscles gradually. Hold each point for 5 seconds at the depth of the muscle tension. Slowly release the pressure. Repeat for the three points on the top of the shoulder with slightly deeper pressure. Use deep breathing to help release tension. As your partner exhales, slowly apply the pressure. During the inhalation, the pressure is gradually released.

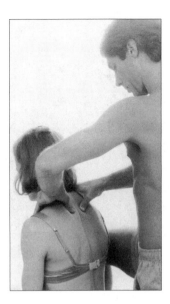

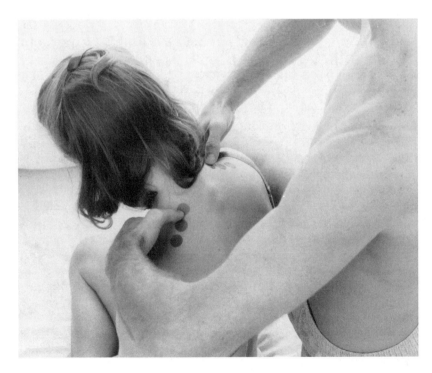

The unconditional love that springs from the heart has both a receptive side— appreciating others as they are and letting them touch us—and an active side—going out to meet, touch, and make contact.

—John Welwood
Challenge of the Heart

61

Behold me here, my love, for I have heard your call across oceans and felt the touch of your wings.

—Kahlil Gibran
A Tear and a Smile

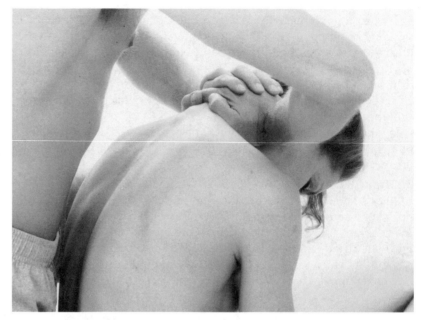

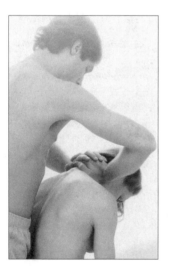

3. Neck Press. Gently push the back of your partner's head forward to expose the back of the neck. Interlace your fingers, and place your palms on either side of your partner's neck. Slowly move your chest closer to your partner's upper back, gradually applying firm pressure to the neck muscles, using the heels of your hands like a clamp. After giving firm compression for about 5 seconds, slowly release the pressure. Slide the heels of your hands to a slightly different area of the neck, and again gradually clamp them inward as your upper body comes closer to your partner. Ask your partner how the amount of pressure feels so that you can adjust it comfortably.

Divide the length of the neck into three sections: upper, middle, and lower. Standing by your partner's left side, place your right hand on the neck with your thumb on the left side and your fingers on the right side. Support your partner's head by holding the forehead with the palm of your left hand as your right hand works on the neck. Begin with the upper section of the neck. Slowly squeeze your fingers toward your thumb like a vise. Press firmly enough that you meet the muscular tension. Hold this level of pressure for a few seconds, and then slowly release it. Slide your hands down to the middle section and gradually reapply the pressure, then go on to the lower section. Repeat this twice more to soften the neck tension. Take care to avoid pressing on the jugular vein in the throat, especially if you are a lot larger than your partner.

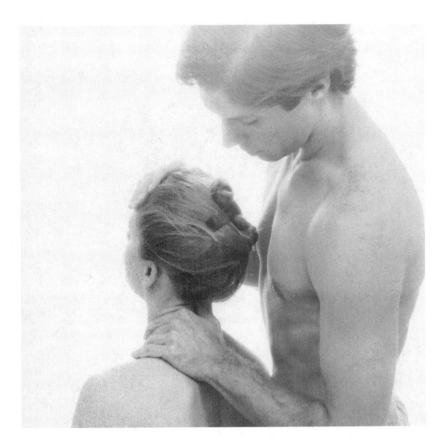

Body touching for both men and women is essential to the truly satisfying love experience. Loving should be harmonious cooperation between men and women in which your hands and every other part of your body gives and receives pleasure.

—Jolan Chang
The Tao of Love and Sex

4. Head Press. Standing by the side of your partner, use your thumb to gradually press into the hollow at the center of the base of the skull (GV 16). Continue to support the forehead with the palm of your other hand. Rotate your thumb clockwise in superslow motion as you gradually apply firm pressure into the hollow and gently tilt the head back for 1 minute.

Press the points underneath the base of the skull as you lift the head upward, giving gentle traction to the neck for approximately 30 seconds. Very gradually release the pressure, bringing the head downward.

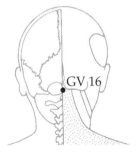

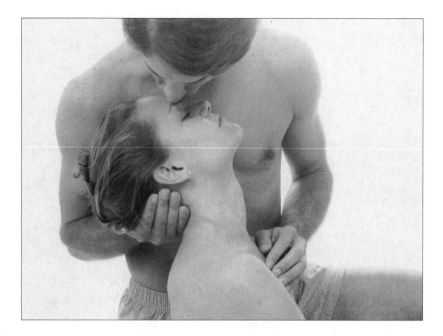

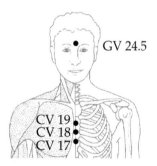

GV 24.5

CV 19
CV 18
CV 17

5. Third Eye Kiss. Position yourself as close as you can by your partner's side. Place one hand over the back of the head. The other hand holds the points on the center of the breastbone (CV 17, 18, 19) using your fingertips. Bend your knees, and kiss the Third Eye point (GV 24.5) in the center of the forehead for 1 minute. As you kiss, create firm suction with your lips. After the Third Eye Kiss, you have several options, depending upon your and your partner's mood:

- **Meditate:** Let your partner simply sit quietly and relax. You may also find it rewarding to meditate immediately after the Third Eye Kiss. Sit next to your partner or back-to-back with your spine straight, close your eyes, and concentrate on your Third Eye point while taking long, slow, deep breaths for 5 to 10 minutes.

- **Hand and Foot Massage:** A wonderful way to finish this shoulder and neck release is to massage your partner's hands and feet. This will rejuvenate your partner, after being so deeply relaxed.

- **Go to Bed Together:** If you and your lover feel like being intimate and relaxing together, take your clothes off and hop into bed. Discover what your partner is like in bed when he or she is under the effect of endorphins, the neurochemicals released as a result of acupressure, which often produce a natural high. Many couples who have taken my training have told me that their acupressure highs are far better than any alcohol or drug they have ever tried.

STRESS REDUCTION POINTS

The acupressure points presented in this section are located in the areas where tension tends to collect. Holding these points on your partner will not only relieve stress but help prevent it from accumulating. Use a combination of steady finger pressure and massage on each point for 1 to 2 minutes.

Familiarize yourself with these points by finding them on your partner's body. Your lover may particularly enjoy having certain points pressed or released. Give these points more attention by massaging and holding them longer, and make them part of your regular routine. You do not have to use all of these points to reduce stress. Holding just a couple of them whenever you and your partner have a few minutes alone together can be effective. Later in this chapter, the Stress Reduction Routine gives a step-by-step sequence for using all these points effectively.

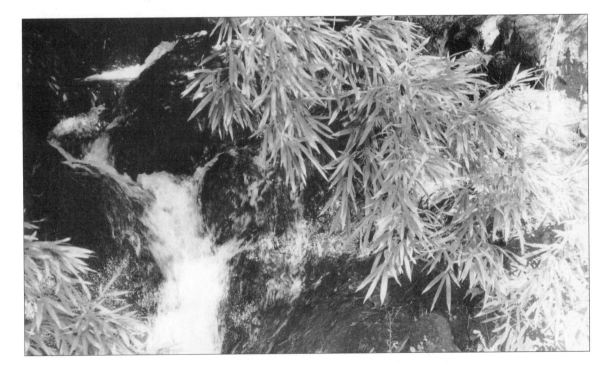

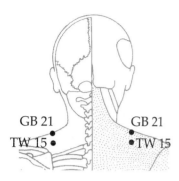

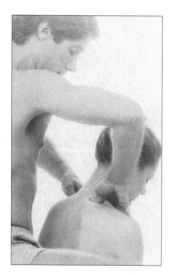

Shoulder Well (GB 21) *and Heavenly Rejuvenation* (TW 15)

Caution: Care must be given to press these points lightly on a pregnant woman. If she is exceptionally physically fit, you can gradually apply more pressure on these shoulder points.

Location: Shoulder Well (GB 21) is on the highest point of the shoulder muscle, one inch out from the base of the neck. Heavenly Rejuvenation (TW 15) is also on the shoulder muscle, one half-inch directly below GB 21.

Benefits: These points commonly get tight, resulting in irritability. It is important for lovers to massage them regularly on each other.

Applications:

While sitting: Stand behind your partner, who is seated in a chair. Rest your fingertips on his or her shoulders for a minute. With your thumbs, gradually make contact with the marble of tension on the top of the shoulders. Hold the point firmly or massage it slowly, firmly kneading the tension out. As you increase the pressure slowly, encourage your partner to breathe deeply. End by holding the point lightly for a minute, then gradually release.

While hugging: Whether you are standing or lying down while hugging, place your inner forearms against your partner's back. Curve your fingers, hooking your fingertips onto the tightest point above the shoulder blades. Gradually apply firm pressure, as you breathe deeply with your partner. After a couple of minutes, slowly release the pressure. End by holding the shoulder points lightly.

For other applications using these acupressure points, see Chapter 8.

Heavenly Pillar (B 10)

Location: One finger-width below the base of the skull, on the ropy muscles one half-inch out from the spine.

Benefits: Pressing this neck point on a regular basis relieves neck tension and helps keep the mind and body in balance.

Applications for Reducing Stress: The best way to use this point is to have your partner lie down on his or her back. Sit close by the top of your partner's head. Gently bring the hair out from underneath the neck, stroking your fingers over the back of the skull.

Sensitively knead the muscles at the back of the neck, squeezing out any tension with your thumbs and fingers in slow motion. Feel for the tightest spot on the upper neck.

Rest the backs of your hands on the ground, and with your fingers curved, support the back of the neck with your fingertips. As you lean against the backs of your hands, slowly straighten your fingers to uplift the neck muscles at the center of the neck. Encourage your partner to breathe deeply in sync with you for 3 minutes. As the muscular tension softens, slowly apply deeper pressure.

To use this point for releasing shoulder and neck tension, see the beginning of this chapter. For other applications, see Chapter 8.

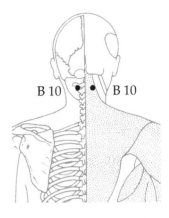

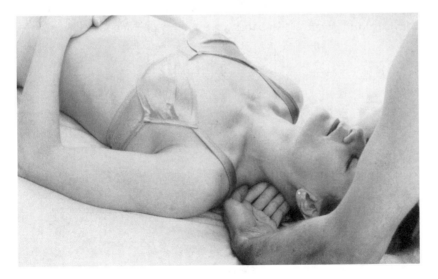

Wind Mansion (GV 16)

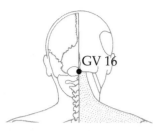

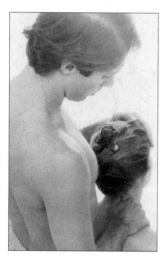

Location: In the center of the back of the head, in the large hollow under the base of the skull (called the medulla).

Benefits: Holding this point opens all the spiritual senses; it is good for the eyes, ears, nose, and throat.

Applications:

With your partner sitting: Stand or kneel behind your partner, who is sitting in a comfortable chair or on a pillow on the floor. Place your thumb in the large hollow under the base of the skull. Place the palm of your other hand on the forehead. Slowly tilt your partner's head back, and gradually apply firm pressure as you rotate the head slowly in one direction and then the other.

With your partner on his or her back: Sit at your partner's head. Place the pads of your middle fingers into the large hollow under the base of your partner's skull. As you apply pressure, slowly pull the head outward toward you, elongating the vertebrae in the neck. Breathe long, slow, deep breaths together in sync, holding the points for 2 or 3 minutes.

While lying on your sides in bed, facing each other: Place your hands on your partner's neck. Using your middle fingers, press the hollow under the base of your partner's skull. Once you feel your middle fingertips fit the hollow area, gradually press upward and slightly outward into the hollow spaces, giving your partner's neck traction.

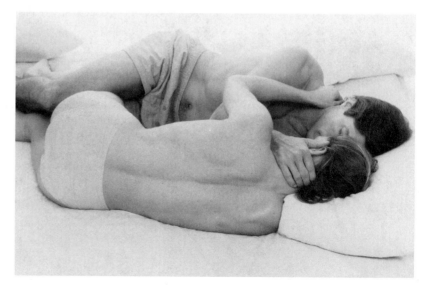

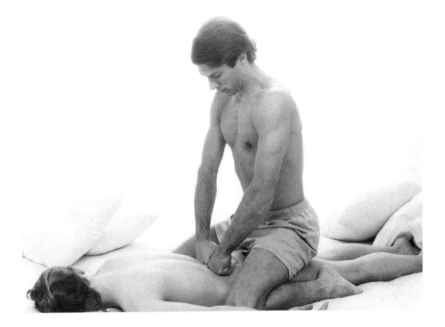

Sea of Vitality (B 23 and B 47)

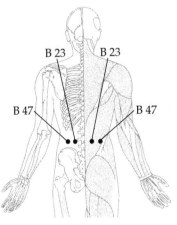

Caution: Do not press on disintegrating disks or fractured or broken bones. If your partner's back is weak, touch these points only lightly, keeping your fingers stationary without exerting pressure. See your doctor first if you have any questions or need medical advice.

Location: In the lower back, two (B 23) and four (B 47) finger-widths out from the spine, at waist level.

Benefits: These are excellent points for relieving and preventing burnout, fatigue, and exhaustion. Use the Sea of Vitality points daily on your partner, especially during stressful times.

Applications:

Standing: Hug your partner, and place your hands on the lower back at waist level. Firmly squeeze the ropelike muscular cords on either side of the spine with your fingertips and the heel of one hand. Place your other hand over that hand for support.

Lying down: Have your partner lie on his or her stomach. Straddle your partner's body near the back of the upper thighs. Gradually apply firm pressure to the Sea of Vitality points, using the backs of your fists in a slow rocking motion and leaning some of the weight of your chest over your fists.

For other ways of using these points, see Chapters 8 and 12.

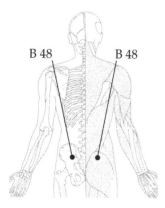

B 48   B 48

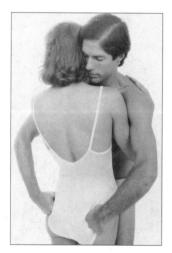

Womb and Vitals (B 48)

Location: One to two finger-widths outside the sacrum (the large bony area at the base of the spine) and midway between the top of the hip bone (iliac crest) and the base of the buttocks.

Benefits: The Womb and Vitals points strongly benefit the sexual-reproductive system. Holding them increases circulation through the pelvis and nurtures the womb and other reproductive organs.

Applications for Relieving Frustration: Every time you grab hold of your partner's "love handles," you instinctively stimulate B 48 with your fingertips. While hugging your partner, either standing up or lying in bed, press these points in the buttocks, using your fingertips. Gradually move closer to your partner's body, and press the outside of your partner's buttocks into the base of the spine at hip level. Since the Womb and Vitals points are located underneath the large buttocks muscles, they often need deeper pressure than your fingers can give. Gradually apply pressure using either the heels of your hands or the knuckles of your fist.

Note: The couple's exercise Riding Your Lover in Chapter 8 also stimulates the Womb and Vitals points.

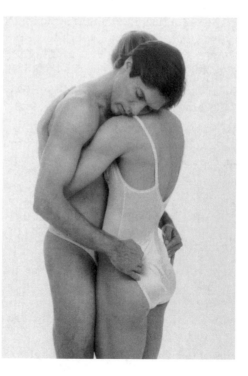

Sacral Points (B 27–B 34)

Location: On the base of the spine, in the hollows of the sacral bone.

Benefits: Holding the Sacral Points can be arousing as well as helpful in relieving your partner's stress, menstrual cramps, and lower back pain. Applying steady firm pressure to these points—which are directly related to the reproductive system—can help overcome impotence.

Applications for Increasing Sexual Energy: Firmly press the slight indentations of your partner's sacral bone while slow dancing or making love. If your partner is lying on his or her belly, you can stimulate these arousal points with the palms of your hands by leaning your body weight to apply pressure.

For intercourse applications using this point, see Chapter 10.

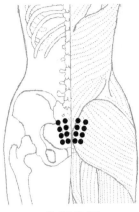

B 27–B 34

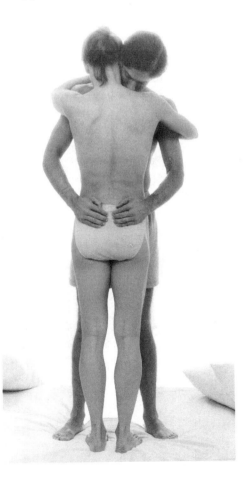

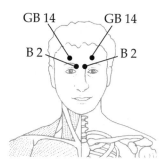

Yang White (GB 14)

Location: On the forehead, one finger-width above the eyebrows, directly above the pupil.

Benefits: Holding this point balances the emotions, clears the mind, improves memory, and reinforces positive thinking.

Applications for Mental Clarity: Lightly touch this point with the soft pads of your fingertips for about a minute as your partner takes a few long deep breaths. You can also kiss your partner gently on this forehead point, at the close of a shoulder and neck massage.

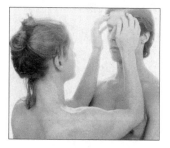

Drilling Bamboo (B 2)

Location: In the indentation of the inner eye socket, where the bridge of the nose meets the ridge of the eyebrows.

Benefits: Holding this point alleviates mental stress and the tensions throughout the forehead that lead to irritability and can sabotage love relationships.

Applications for Relieving Stress: After hugging your partner in a standing position, gently place your thumbs on the Drilling Bamboo points. Let the weight of your partner's head come forward onto your thumbs, or else let the weight of your hands lean into these stress reduction points. Do not press with force; instead, use your body weight or your partner's.

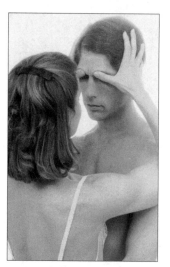

When your partner is sitting comfortably in a chair: Stand close by his or her left side. Bend your knees, and use the palm of your right hand to support the back of your partner's head. Place the thumb and index finger of your left hand on the Drilling Bamboo points, and gradually apply pressure, holding for at least 1 minute while you both breathe deeply together.

The Drilling Bamboo points are excellent for releasing general daily stress. Incorporate this last technique at the end of the shoulder and neck massage. On using this point during intercourse, see Chapter 10.

Elegant Mansion (K 27)

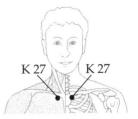

Location: In the depression directly below the protrusions of the collarbones.

Benefits: This is a valuable point for rejuvenating the immune system during stressful times or after a long day.

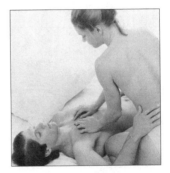

Applications for Rejuvenation: Have your partner lie down on his or her back. Either sit close on one side, or straddle your partner's waist. Place your thumbs a couple of inches below the throat, in the hollow areas directly below the heads of the collarbone. Slowly lean some of the weight of your chest into your thumbs, gradually applying firm steady pressure. Coach your partner to breathe deeply into the Elegant Mansion point while the pressure is being applied to it. Breathe deeply in sync while you hold the points for about 2 minutes.

This is a powerful point to press after giving your partner the Shoulder and Neck Massage.

Sea of Tranquility (CV 17)

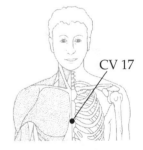

Location: On the center of the breastbone, four finger-widths up from the base of the bone.

Benefits: Holding this point opens the heart's chamber inside the chest and increases emotional intimacy.

Applications for Emotional Balancing: With your fingertips, firmly hold the indentations on the center of the breastbone at the level of the heart. Hold for at least a minute as you and your partner synchronize breathing deeply together.

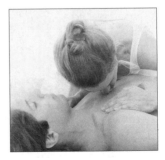

A full-body hug is the most powerful way to stimulate this wonderful calming point. Fitting your breastbones together like puzzle pieces during a full-body hug presses the Sea of Tranquility point, opening a satisfying warmth into both of your hearts.

Another alternative is to take off your partner's shirt and kiss and suck the Sea of Tranquility point. After your lips stimulate this point, hug your partner with affection and breathe deeply in sync as a romantic way to begin lovemaking.

For using this point in other love positions, see Chapters 8 and 10.

Bigger Stream (K 3)

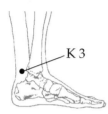

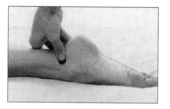

Caution: Although this point can promote fertility and help a woman get pregnant, it should be held only gently after the third month of pregnancy to calm the fetus.

Location: In the back of the ankle, midway between the inside anklebone and the Achilles tendon.

Benefits: Holding these ankle points with the Sea of Vitality points (B 23 and B 47) in the lower back (see Chapter 13) can balance either an excess or a lack of sexual desire.

Applications for Relaxation:

With your partner sitting in a chair: Kneel or sit on the floor close to your partner's feet. Place your thumbs on these inner ankle points with your fingers on the outside of the ankles. Squeeze between the anklebones and the Achilles tendon. Hold for at least a minute, leaning your body weight toward the feet.

With your partner lying down on his or her stomach: Place your thumbs on the Bigger Stream points. Place your other fingers on the outside of the ankle. Squeeze between the anklebone and the Achilles tendon as you lean some of your weight downward to apply pressure. Hold for 1 to 2 minutes, leaning your body weight into your hands.

Try kissing and sucking on the Bigger Stream point during foreplay. After a foot massage, use your mouth to stimulate the point, then slowly kiss your way up the inner parts of the leg.

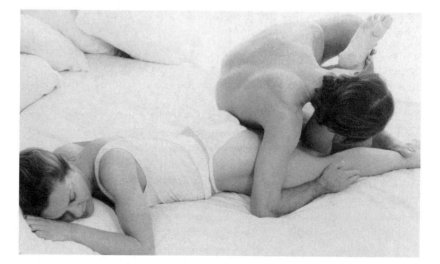

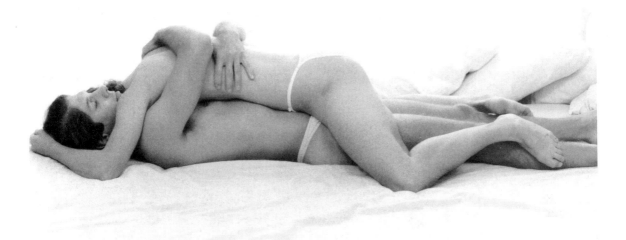

Grandparent-Grandchild (Sp 4)

Location: In the upper arch of the foot, one thumb-width from the ball of the foot.

Benefits: Holding this point fosters emotional stability, trust, and a sense of security in a love relationship.

Applications for Rejuvenation and Sensuality: The foot is one of the most wonderful areas of the body to massage. After a long day on your feet, a foot massage can completely rejuvenate you. An erotic foot massage given with the spirit of love can arouse a wonderful sexual connection. See Chapter 8 for instructions on how to massage your partner's feet.

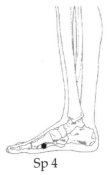

Sp 4

When you are lying front-to-front in bed together with your clothes off, make contact with the arches of your feet against your partner's legs using your insteps and toes. Slide your feet over your partner's legs, creating an energetic circuit throughout your bodies. Sensually stroking each other's legs with your arches stimulates the Grandparent-Grandchild points, energizing your relationship's sexual dimension.

The Lovemaking Progressions in Chapter 10 will show you how to incorporate this erotic technique while making love.

STRESS REDUCTION ROUTINE

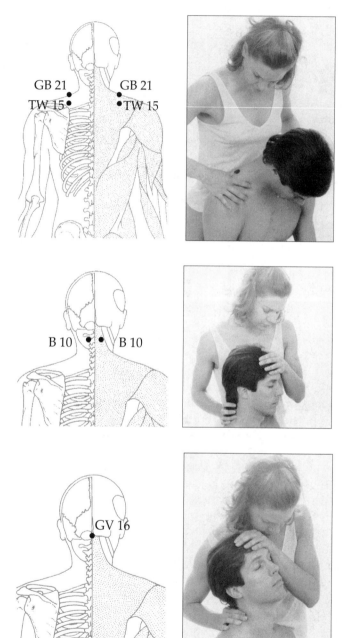

Before you give your partner this relaxing acupressure massage, ask that he or she refresh in the bathroom. While your partner is washing his or her face, select a comfortable chair that has a medium to low back, and position the chair so that you have room to stand behind it. Have your partner sit down comfortably, with his or her back firmly supported.

Remember to apply pressure gradually. Ask your partner to close his or her eyes and begin deep breathing. Also ask for feedback on areas that feel good that your partner would like you to focus on more, tight or sore areas that need less pressure, and areas that need deeper pressure. Spend approximately 1 minute on each of the following steps. Feel free to improvise based on your partner's feedback as well as your own intuition.

Begin with your partner in a sitting position.

1. Knead the Shoulder Muscles (GB 21, TW 15). Do this in slow motion.

2. Massage the Neck (B 10). Start by standing to the side of your partner. Place your palm on your partner's forehead for support. Press and knead your partner's shoulder and neck muscles, using your fingers on one side and your thumb on the other.

3. Gradually Press Wind Mansion (GV 16). With your thumb, press into the large hollow in the center of the base of the skull, as your other hand continues to hold the forehead.

Ask your partner to lie down on his or her stomach.

4. Knead the Lower Back (B 23, B 47). Straddle your partner's body near the back of his or her upper thighs. Slowly knead the lower back muscles with your hands. Then use the backs of your fists in a slow, rocking motion, leaning some of your weight over your fists.

5. Knead the Buttocks (B 48). Grasp the muscles in your partner's buttocks and knead them like pizza dough. Then rock the backs of your fists over the buttocks as you lean some of your weight into the musculature.

6. Sacral Press (B 27–B 34). With the heels of your hands, apply pressure to the base of your partner's spine. Lean most of the weight of your upper body into the heels of your hands, firmly pressing the sacral points as you encourage your partner to breathe deeply.

Ask your partner to turn over onto his or her back, and sit at his or her side.

7. Lightly Touch the Forehead (GB 14, B 2). With your partner's eyes closed, lightly touch the center of the forehead. With your other hand, gently touch the Drilling Bamboo (B 2) point, in the slight indentation of the upper ridge of the eye where the bridge of the nose meets the eye socket.

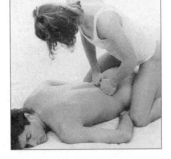

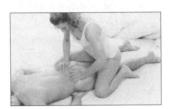

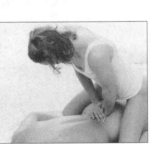

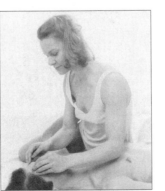

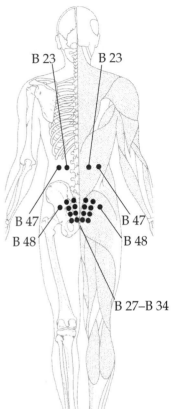

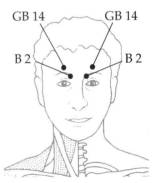

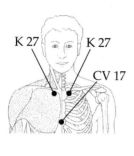

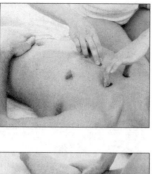

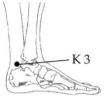

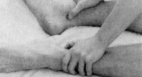

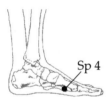

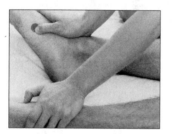

Inside of Foot

8. Chest Press (K 27, CV 17). With one hand, hold the indentations directly below your partner's collarbones, using your thumb on one side and your index or middle finger on the other. With the fingertips of your other hand, hold the indentations on the center of your partner's breastbone.

9. Ankle Press (K 3). Move down your partner's body to his or her feet, pressing the Bigger Stream points on both of the Achilles tendons and ankles. Lean most of your weight into your partner's body as you squeeze K 3 with your thumbs. Breathe deeply as you hold these ankle points for 1 minute.

10. Arch of Foot Massage (Sp 4). While sitting at your partner's feet, thoroughly massage the arch of his or her foot and all the toes. End by grasping all the toes firmly for 1 minute. Then very slowly release the pressure, leaving your partner in a deep state of relaxation.

SUPPORT YOUR PARTNER

The following couple's exercises gently stretch the muscles and stimulate acupressure points through satisfying body contact and slow graceful movements. As you practice these exercises, focus on breathing deeply into your belly to open sexual energy for making love.

Back-and-Forth Embrace

1. Sit on a rug or on your bed with your bodies close together. Wrap your legs and arms around each other.
2. Slowly rock your bodies back and forth.
3. Let your head go with the movement. Create a rhythm for deep breathing: Inhale as your head and body come backward, and exhale as your head and body come forward.
4. Continue for at least a few minutes.

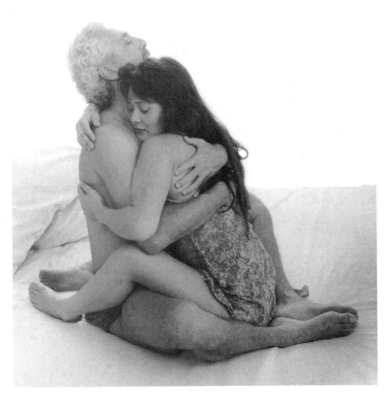

Many men and women mistakenly believe that if they experience their sexual energy, they must do something about it— they must perform, act it out, discharge it. Since having sexual energy is simply a function of being alive, all they need to do with it is experience it. They can learn to contain it and allow it to spread out to the whole body rather than to express it genitally.

—Jack Lee Rosenberg

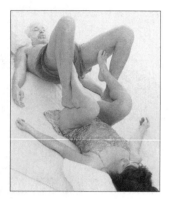

Thigh Bridge

1. Lie down on your backs with your heads positioned in opposite directions and your buttocks almost touching.

2. Both of you place the soles of your feet on the backs of each other's thighs. Take turns arching the pelvis upward by pressing your feet against each other's thighs.

3. Scoot your bodies as close together as possible.

4. Inhale as you press your feet against the back of your partner's thighs and bridge upward; exhale as you come downward. Continue for about a minute.

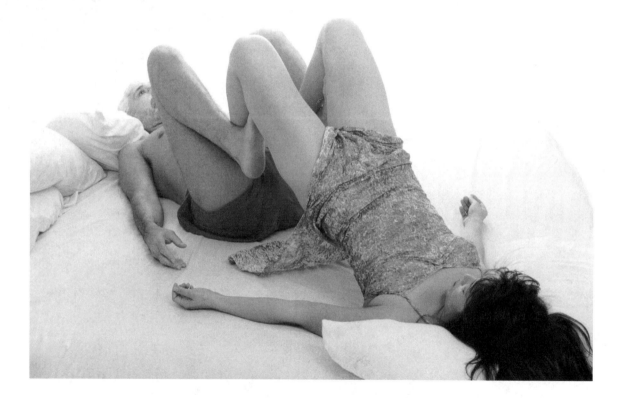

Double Butterfly

1. Remain on your backs, in the same position as in the Thigh Bridge. Place the bottoms of your feet together on your partner's belly.

2. The partner with the most flexibility should position his or her legs underneath.

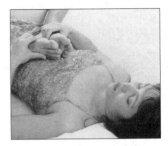

3. Place your hands on your partner's feet. Close your eyes and give your partner a wonderful foot massage.

4. Complete this couple's exercise by lightly stroking your partner's feet up toward the ankles and calf muscles as far as your hands can comfortably reach. Breathe deeply, and enjoy the pleasurable sensations.

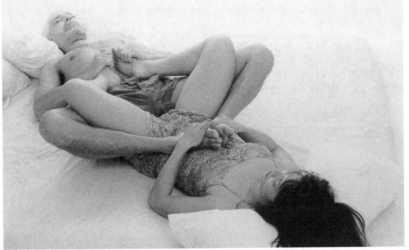

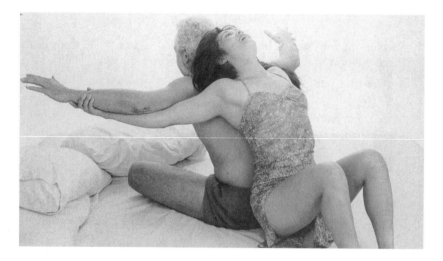

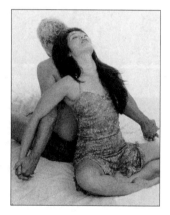

Loving Back-to-Back

This seesaw exercise adds flexibility to your spine and opens the chest, increasing the energy flow between you and your lover.

Caution: People with severe back problems may not be able to practice this exercise. If your partner is stiff or has had a past back problem, use care when leaning back.

1. Sit back-to-back. Reach backward to hold hands with your partner.

2. Slowly rock your bodies back and forth.

Suggestions

- **Breathe with the Movement:** Inhale as your body comes back; exhale as your body moves forward.

- **Leg Stretch:** Bringing your legs straight out in front of you will give you an excellent stretch in the backs of your legs, especially when your partner leans on your back.

Advanced Variations

- **Arching on Your Partner's Back:** Hold hands, or link your arms together at the elbows. While you bend your knees, with feet flat on the floor, your partner can extend his or her legs straight out. As you lean back, slowly raise your pelvis upward. Your partner can signal how much weight is enough. Then lower your buttocks to the ground, sliding your feet straight out in front of you. Your partner then bends his or her legs, slowly arching up onto your back. Repeat several times, inhaling up and exhaling forward.

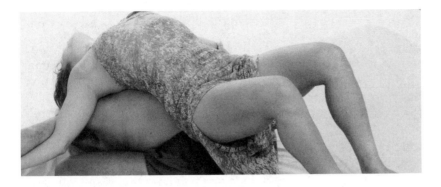

- **Reaching Up and Over:** As you lean back, lifting your pelvis up, stretch your arms up and back. This will give you and your partner another powerful full-body stretch.

- **Draping the Body over the Back:** Kneel, while your partner remains sitting, immediately regaining back-to-back contact. Now, reach back, holding your partner's hand or interlacing your fingers. Slowly rock back and forth as you breathe deeply. To increase the power of the stretch, gradually bring your arms up overhead. As you lean forward, bringing your arms forward, you will pull your partner over your back. Continue to breathe deeply together, moving slowly into each stretch without straining.

ACUPRESSURE POINTS

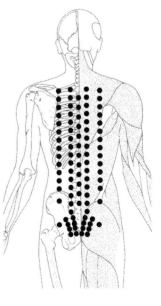

Sacral Points: These are used for sexual reproduction problems, such as impotence, vaginal discharge, and genital pain.

Mid-spinal Region Points: These can open your heart and soul as well as relieve anxiety, back pain, and stiffness.

Internal Organ-associated Points: These benefit the functioning of the organs and the nervous system.

Back Muscle Points: These prevent and relieve back spasms and pain, neck problems, headaches, sciatica, and calf cramps.

Benefits: Loving Back-to-Back strengthens the central nervous system and can avert a variety of back problems, including sciatica, lumbago, and spinal stiffness. This exercise can enable you and your partner to live healthier, longer lives.

The Double Hug

There's no feeling more secure than that of being held by your partner. There is also nothing more liberating than breathing deeply with the person you love. The Double Hug provides a full-body mutual embrace, merging two souls into one.

The following instructions are for both partners to follow simultaneously:

1. Sit cross-legged, side by side, facing in opposite directions, with your right thighs together.
2. Bring your left leg straight out, or bend your left leg outward, with your left heel beside your left buttock.
3. As you lean toward your partner, raise your left hand up and embrace, with your head over your partner's left shoulder.
4. Adjust your bodies to have maximum contact, closeness, and comfort.

In embracing unconditional love you surrender all emotions and thoughts that separate you from well-being and harmony. This is the essential commitment in transformation and it must be renewed every day. Love is a daily celebration of aliveness and permission to go deeper.

—Richard Moss, M.D.
The I That Is We

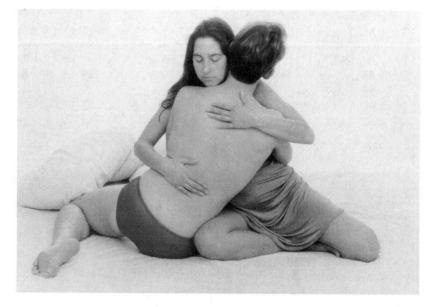

Suggestions

- Close your eyes and breathe long, slow, deep breaths into each other's ears. Hold your breath for a few seconds at the top of each inhalation. Let the sound of your partner's breath stimulate you to breathe slowly and deeply. The longer you can stay in sync with each other's breath, the more powerful your experience will be together. Stimulating each other to breathe will charge your bodies with a tremendous amount of energy.

- Continue to breathe deeply together into each other's ears. After a while, slowly move the upper part of your bodies in a large graceful circle. Once enough energy has been generated from breathing together and you have surrendered your mind to this incredibly vital force, your bodies will begin moving together spontaneously. This deep breathing ritual creates an altered state and can be a powerful transformational tool for healing yourselves and heightening your sexual relationship.

Variations

- **Back Massage:** As you embrace, try massaging each other's backs. Curve your fingertips to firmly knead any tight back muscles.

- **Back and Neck Massage:** Holding your right hand on the lower back, your left hand massages your partner's neck. Feel free to ask your partner for feedback about whether to touch more lightly or more firmly. Enjoy the feeling of touching and being touched.

- **Throat Hug:** Lift your chins upward, gently touching throat-to-throat. Adjust your head and body until they fit together comfortably. Then gradually increase the strength of your embrace until you feel a passionate connection.

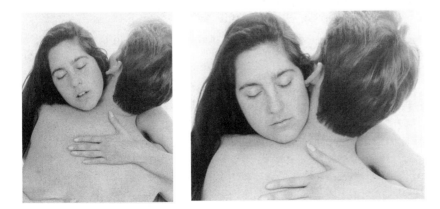

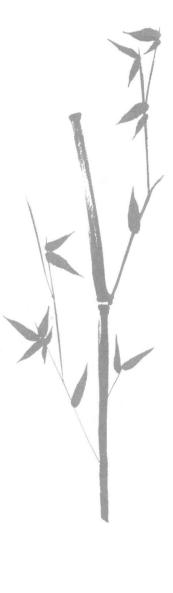

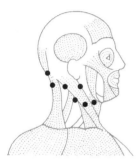

Windows of the Sky

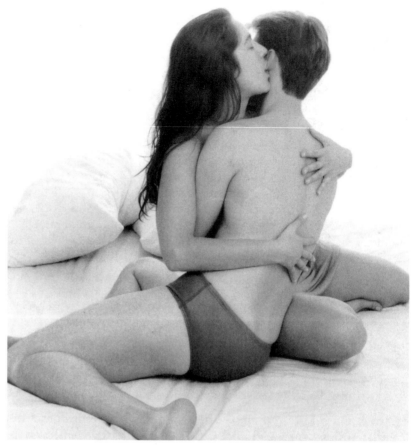

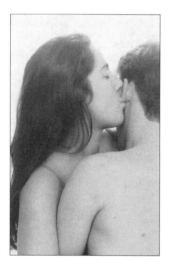

- **Kissing the Windows of the Sky:** If the spirit moves you, stimulate the points on your partner's neck by kissing, sucking, or licking. Then return to breathing into your partner's ear.

- **Hot, Wet Ear Massage:** There are more than 150 points in each ear— so many points in so little space that no matter where you touch or kiss the ear, you will be stimulating points. While you embrace your partner in your arms, breathe slowly and deeply into the ear, creatively using your tongue on all of these ear points.

Benefits: The deep breathing in this position charges your bodies with the life force. As you hold the acupressure points in this embrace, powerful healing energy circulates, nurturing your individual vital systems as well as your love relationship.

The Double Hug posture opens the neck and throat, which is a bridge between the mind and body as well as a powerful communication center. By practicing this posture regularly, you and your partner create an intimate, vulnerable connection, enabling you to express emotions more freely.

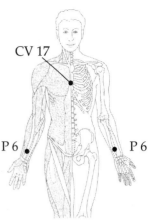

Acupressure Points

Point	Name	Location
P 6	*Inner Gate*	Three finger-widths above the center of the inner wrist crease
CV 17	*Sea of Tranquility*	On the center of the breastbone, four finger-widths up from the base of the breastbone
B 10	*Heavenly Pillar*	One finger-width below the base of the skull on the ropy muscles, one-half inch outward from the spine
SI 10	*Shoulder Blade*	Where the humerus (upper arm bone) meets the scapula (shoulder blade), below the acromion
B 38	*Vital Diaphragm*	Between the shoulder blades and the spine, at the level of the heart
B 23, B 47	*Sea of Vitality*	On the lower back, two and four finger-widths away from the spine at waist level, in line with the belly button

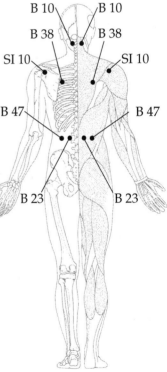

SPIRITUAL ATTUNEMENT

The following routine can become a sacred ritual for sharing powerful full-body experiences and each other's innermost feelings. It begins by releasing each other's stress and culminates in a deeply harmonious full-body embrace.

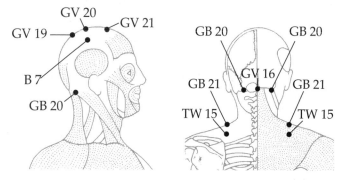

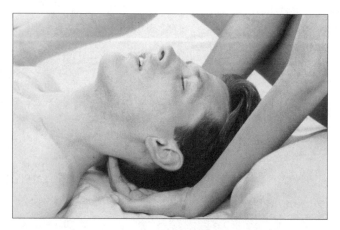

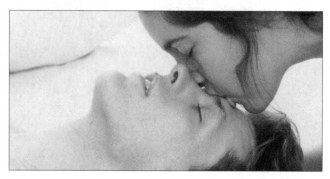

Sit on a pillow at your partner's head as your partner lies on his or her back.

1. Massage the Shoulders. Place your hands on your partner's shoulders. Sensually move your hands in slow motion, kneading any tension out of the shoulder muscles as you press points GB 21 and TW 15.

2. Ease Your Partner's Mental Stress. Place your fingertips on the Gates of Consciousness point (GB 20), underneath the base of your partner's skull on both sides. Fit your fingertips into the indentations underneath the skull, allowing the weight of your partner's head to rest on your fingertips. As you hold these points, gradually pull the head outward to apply traction, and hold for 2 minutes or until you feel a pulsation on both sides. Then bring your middle fingers into the center of the base of the skull, and press Wind Mansion (GV 16), giving the neck traction.

3. Sensually Rake the Skull. With your fingers curved, slowly caress the back of your partner's head with your fingertips, moving from the base of the skull up behind the ears to the top of the head. Be careful not to pull the hair. Repeat this stroke a few times. Then place your thumbs on the top of your partner's head to press GV 19, GV 20, GV 21, and B 7. Massage the skull in slow motion with your fingertips as your thumbs hold these points.

4. Kiss the Third Eye. With your fingers curved, place your fingertips underneath the base of the skull, and again gradually pull your partner's head outward. As you give traction, lean forward to kiss the center of the forehead with the inner wet portion of your lips. Give your partner's Third Eye point (GV 24.5) firm suction as you breathe deeply for 2 minutes. Then, slowly, move over to sit by your lover's side.

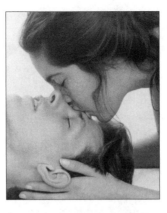

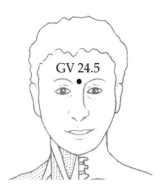

5. Final Balancing. Place one hand lightly on the back of the top of your partner's head (GV 20, GV 21), using all of your fingertips. With the third fingertip of your other hand, gently hold the Third Eye point (GV 24.5). Breathe deeply with your partner, focusing your attention on the Third Eye point for at least a minute. This strongly opens the point and as a result can increase your intuition. As you continue to hold the top of the head, move your other hand off the Third Eye point and down to the center of the breastbone (CV 17), the Sea of Tranquility point. Then gently place the center of your forehead on your partner's third eye area. Close your eyes, and breathe slowly and deeply in sync with each other to develop your spiritual intimacy.

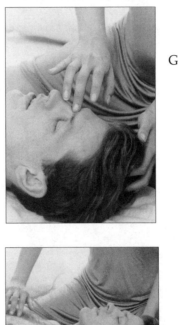

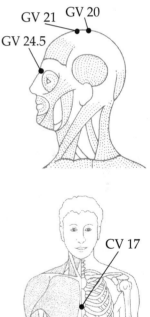

HARMONY BONDING: A TANTRIC EMBRACE

Let us unite, let us

hold each other tightly,

let us merge our hearts . . .

—Nikos Kazantzakis

This following whole-body embrace can be a nurturing, healing, daily sexual practice. Intercourse is not necessary for engaging in this wonderful Tantric embrace.

Either partner can be on top. The man's penis can be either up on the woman's belly, limp and hanging downward, or erect and inside her vagina. If both partners feel good about his being inside, they will use a minimum amount of movement, just enough to maintain his erection.

Completely embrace each other, with your legs intertwined and your feet touching your partner's feet. The palms of your hands are touching your partner's palms, and your fingers are interlaced; or you can just wrap your arms around each other. Lift your chins, placing your throats together, or kiss each other. Try to connect all parts of your body, from head to toe, as you embrace. Lie as still as possible to rejuvenate and heal your nervous systems. Consciously breathe slowly and deeply together, opening your bodies' life forces to flow, merge, and harmonize.

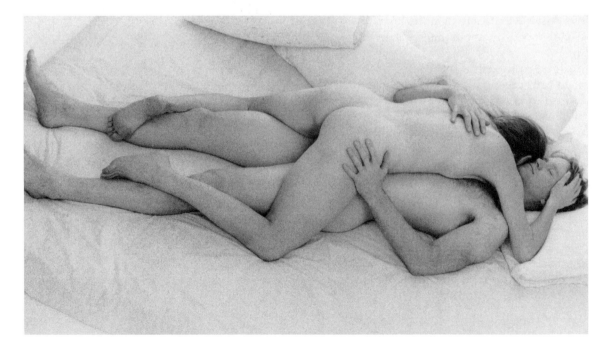

Chapter 6

AROUSING A WOMAN

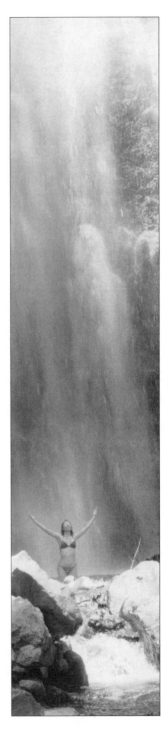

*T*his chapter provides detailed instructions and guidelines for fully arousing a woman, whether by a man or
another woman. First you will learn how to give an
erotic full-body acupressure massage. Then you will explore six sets
of arousal points for women. The chapter ends by describing an
arousal routine using each of these points for stimulating, nurturing,
and satisfying a woman.

More than four thousand years ago in ancient China, the Yellow
Emperor commissioned his ministers to study the best ways to live a
long and healthy life. He was particularly interested in knowing how
to cultivate, sustain, and transform sexual energy. His greatest adviser
on the secrets of sex was known as the Plain Girl.

The Plain Girl taught the Yellow Emperor that a man's sexual
responses are simple compared with the depth and complexity of a
woman's. To arouse and satisfy a woman completely, she taught him,
it is essential for a man to breathe consciously, slowly, and deeply and
to reduce the speed of his movements until they are gradual and
graceful. If he can envision each of his caresses unfolding in
superslow motion as he breathes slowly and deeply, staying present
with her responses, he can fully embrace her sensual delights and
give her complete satisfaction.

FULL-BODY MASSAGE

The following instructions guide both men and women to touch and
massage a woman's body in a deeply erotic way. If you, the massager,
become aroused during this routine it is essential to slow down your
breathing and your hand movements, allowing time for the woman's
sexual desire to grow. Your intention to be affectionate, intimate, and
fully present with her can create an openness for sexual energy to
emerge and flow.

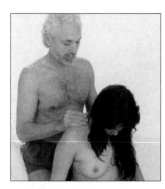

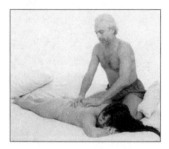

Begin by massaging all parts of her body. When a woman's whole body is touched, she feels profoundly nurtured and loved. Her body circuitry opens to greater pleasure, cultivating a whole-body orgasm as opposed to a localized genital orgasm. Encourage her to breathe deeply, to relax completely, and to receive fully the gifts and pleasures of your touch.

Massage oil or lotion is optional; ask your partner what she prefers. Use oils or lotions that are not irritating to the vaginal membrane. Before you begin, be sure that the room is warm and free of drafts.

1. **Ask your partner to take a comfortable sitting position.** Massage her shoulders and neck. Knead the muscles in superslow motion, asking her how much pressure feels best. Breathe deeply, and keep your own spine fairly straight, neither twisted nor slumped.

2. **Have your partner lie down on her stomach.** You may want to place a pillow under her chest for her breasts and another under her hips. Work your way slowly down her back, and then massage her sacrum and buttocks. Be open to feedback such as "more slowly please," "a little less hard," or "move up a bit higher."

3. **Very slowly glide your hands over her legs,** and massage her feet, spending time touching all parts of each toe.

You can enjoy your partner's body with your hands and your lips and your tongue. Not only her looks but her smell and the feel of her skin has its own sensuous pleasure. Caressing her body's sensitive areas will arouse her.

—Jolan Chang
The Tao of Love and Sex

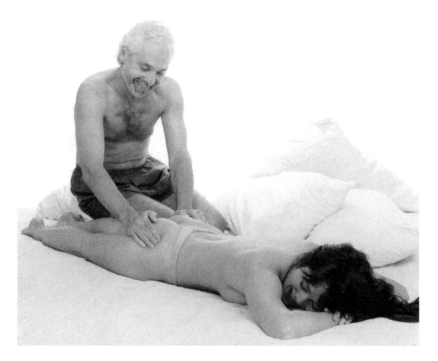

4. **Turn her over on her back.** Slowly stroke your way up her legs. Tantalize her genitals—come close, lightly graze them, but deliberately move on. Gently caress the sides of her body up to her breasts, allowing your fingers to glide lightly over her nipples. Then massage her shoulders, kneading the muscles like bread.

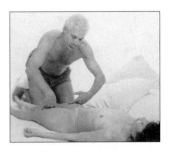

5. **Lightly stroke down the inside of her arms** through the center of her palms. If she responds with deep breathing or sighing, repeat this light stroke on the inside of her arms a few more times.

6. **After lovingly massaging her hands,** glide up her arms to her breasts. Enjoy gently touching her breasts and nipples.

7. **Spend some time caressing her breasts.** Encircle the nipples to stimulate the acupressure point Center of the Breasts (St 17) with your fingertips. Gently roll the nipples back and forth between your thumbs and fingers.

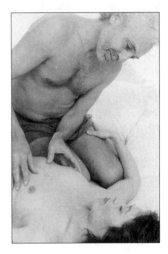

8. **Slowly slide your hands down your partner's body,** placing the palm of one hand between the navel and pubic bone. Gradually apply firm pressure to the Sea of Intimacy points (CV 2–CV 6).

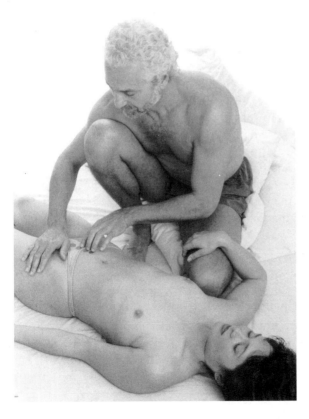

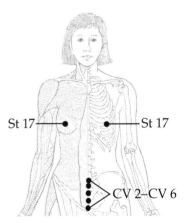

In order to live a harmonious and creative life, you need to have both your inner female and male energies fully developed and functioning correctly together. To fully integrate the inner male and female, you need to put the female in the guiding position. This is her natural function. She is your intuition....

—Shakti Gawain
Living in the Light

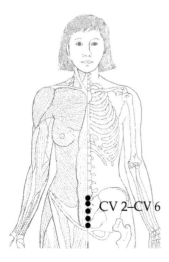

CV 2–CV 6

9. **Tantalize her sexuality by lightly stroking up the inner thigh** and slowly exploring the genital area with your other hand for a few minutes. Caress your partner's precious gate, gradually approaching the opening. Enjoy fondling her lips and feeling her moistness for a couple of minutes. Explore the inner lips of her vagina and the opening of the vaginal wall.

10. **Slowly bring your index and middle fingertips into her vagina,** with the pads of your fingers facing upward. Gently make small, slow circular motions, lightly touching the roof of the vagina for a while.

    A couple of inches inside the roof of the vagina is rippled tissue called the G spot—short for Grafenberg or, in Tantric circles, for Goddess. Stroking this area can greatly deepen a woman's sexual response.

    Consider the vagina a universe, containing a multitude of stars. The vagina has numerous acupressure points, varying in location from woman to woman. Discovering the sacred map of your lover's universe is exciting and rewarding.

11. **With your fingers extended fully inside the vagina,** slowly stroke the pads of your fingertips over the vaginal roof by curving your fingers. Continue to repeat this "come here" hand gesture inside the vagina as you encourage her to breathe slowly and deeply with you. Ask her to give you feedback about the pressure and speed of your finger movements.

12. **Gradually apply pressure to the Sea of Intimacy points** (CV 2–CV 6) in the lower belly, with the whole palm of your other hand. Encourage her to breathe deeply into her belly. If she feels comfortable with firmer abdominal pressure, increase your palm pressure slowly toward your fingertips, inside the vagina. As you direct the pressure of your palm on the belly and your fingertips inside the vagina gradually toward each other, ask your partner for feedback, and breathe deeply together.

13. **With the fingers inside the vagina,** slowly apply pressure on the vaginal roof. Direct the pressure toward the palm of your outside hand. As you breathe deeply, imagine your hands creating a powerful direct connection deep inside your partner's womb.

14. **Explore holding the clitoris lightly,** keeping your fingers still. Encourage your partner to breathe deeply and to move freely against your fingers in ways most pleasurable to her. This also enables you to know what areas, angles, pressures, and movements are most arousing for her.

After a while, you both may want to have intercourse. Simply ask her. If words seem unnecessary, go with your intuition. Enjoy each moment, communicating your love through the quality of your touch.

Rather than making love, a secure embrace with contact from head to toe is sometimes all that needs to happen. Holding each other's bodies creates a sacred space that does not have to be filled with anything—not talking, not even an arousing touch. When you feel your bodies fit together, simply hold each other and breathe deeply in sync. Embracing from head to toe connects many acupressure points and increases the healing contact. The stillness of the embrace encourages the life force to flow from point to point throughout your bodies, creating a deep and transcendent experience.

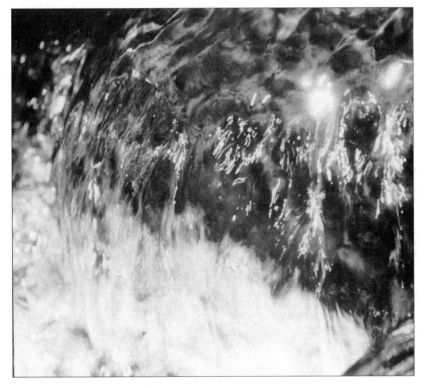

Women relate intimacy to the heart or the soul more than to the brain or the genitals, although when true sexual intimacy does occur, sexual passion is its by-product. This seems to be true in all areas, not just sex.

—Charles and Caroline Muir
Tantra: The Art of Conscious Loving

SIX SETS OF AROUSAL POINTS
FOR WOMEN

This section contains six sets of acupressure points, giving you the location and some applications for each point. Any combination of these points can be used to begin an erotic journey. At the end of this section, the Arousal Routine for Women will show you how to use these points in a step-by-step sequence.

Hidden Clarity (Sp 1) *and Great Sincerity* (Lv 1)

Location: At the base of the nail of the large toe, on the outer and inner corners.

Benefits: Holding these points calms the spirit and clears the brain.

Applications for Arousal: After taking a bath or shower, the best way to arouse these points is to suck on the large toe. A little nibbling is fine, but sucking goes a long way. This can be especially arousing to a woman; try it as a prelude to making love.

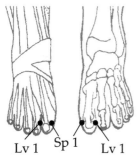

Lv 1 Sp 1 Lv 1

Top Front of Feet

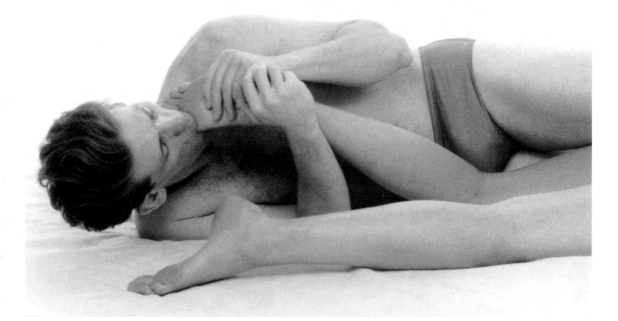

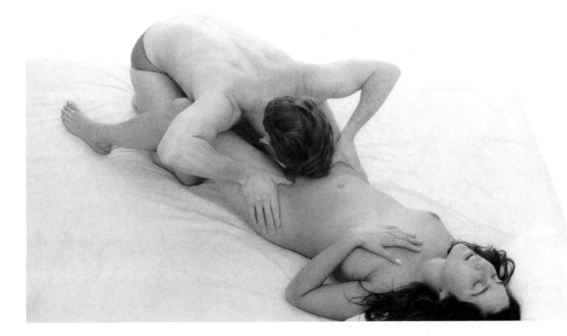

Rushing Door (Sp 12) *and Mansion Cottage* (Sp 13)

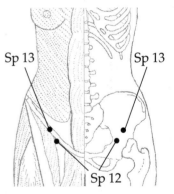

Location: In the pelvic area, in the middle of the crease where the leg joins the trunk of the body.

Benefits: Holding these points particularly increases a woman's sexual response and enhances sensations in the genitals.

Applications for Arousal: With your partner lying on her back, kneel between her legs. Gently place the heel of your hands on the groin crease where her thigh joins the trunk of her body. With your fingers lightly on her belly, slowly lean some of the weight of your chest into your partner's groin points, gradually increasing the pressure. Adjust your hands for your comfort, and hold for 2 minutes while breathing deeply.

Grasping the pelvis while holding these points can be incredibly arousing for both intercourse and oral sex. Firmly hold your partner's pelvis, bringing the palms of your hands to the base of her hip bone. Rotate your thumbs until they find the thick, taut, ropy band in the groin, halfway between the hip bone and the tip of the pubic bone. As you grasp hold of the pelvis in this way, passionately pull your partner's body toward you.

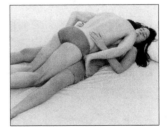

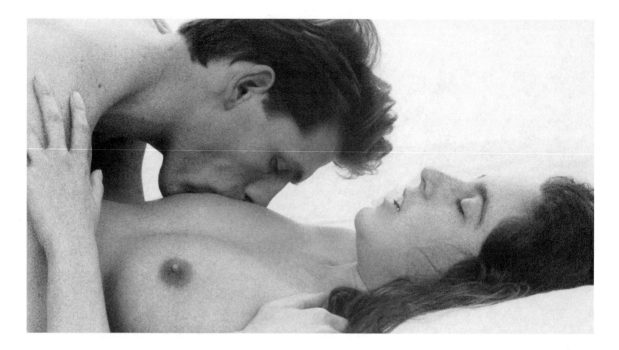

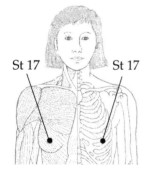

St 17   St 17

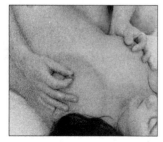

Center of the Breasts (St 17)

Location: In the center of the nipple.

Benefits: Touching these points arouses a woman's sexual energy, providing a strong oral and genital connection. Both acupressurists and acupuncturists are forbidden to use these points professionally.

Applications for Arousal: Slowly and gently roll the nipple between your thumb and index finger. You can gradually increase the pressure, but be careful not to hurt your partner. Nipple sensitivity varies, and you need to ask your partner to signal or tell you before you squeeze too hard. Nothing ruins a mood or breaks your partner's trust in you more quickly than an insensitive, hurtful nipple twist.

Another excellent way to stimulate this arousal point is to kiss and gently suck it. Imagine you are sucking a straw full of a delicious thick chocolate milkshake or that you are a baby sucking your mother's milk. Concentrate on breathing deeply as you suck. Then with the tip of your tongue, circle the nipple slowly. Alternate sucking and circling the nipple with your tongue, and continue to breathe deeply.

Human Welcome (St 9) *and Water Rushing* (St 10)

Location: On the side of the throat. *Caution:* Do not press these points strongly. Never apply pressure to both sides at the same time since these points lie on a major artery.

Benefits: Touching these points particularly heightens a woman's erotic experience.

Applications for Arousal: Few words are needed to describe how to use these highly vulnerable, sensual points. Simply kiss and suck them to arouse your partner's passion.

A Spiritual Note: Ancient Chinese sexology teaches that stimulating these points on the neck enhances a man's and woman's harmony with the natural forces of heaven and earth.

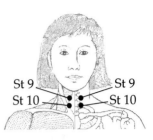

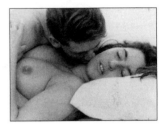

Sacral Points (B 27–B 34)

Location: On the base of the spine, in the hollows of the sacral bone.

Benefits: Holding these points firmly for at least a minute significantly increases a woman's sexual pleasure.

Applications: With your fingertips, feel for the slight indentations in the sacral bone, while slow dancing or making love. If your partner is lying on her belly, stimulate these arousal points with the palms of your hands by leaning some of your body weight over your palms. Stimulating these points is excellent both during foreplay and while giving your lover a massage. Pressing them can greatly heighten a woman's pleasure during both intercourse and oral sex.

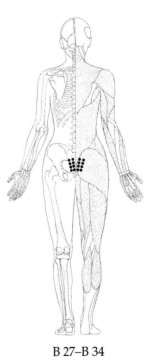

B 27–B 34

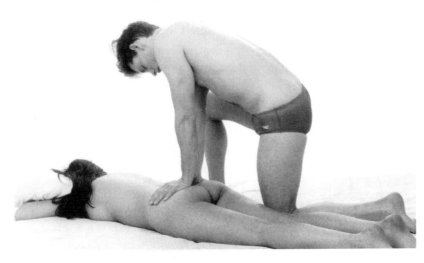

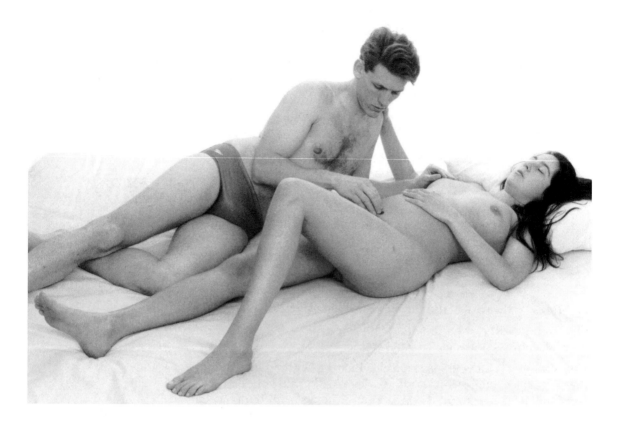

Gate of Origin (CV 4)

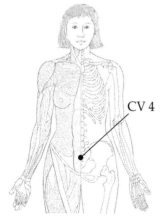

CV 4

Location: Four finger-widths below the belly button.

Benefits: Touching this lower abdominal point heightens a woman's sexual awareness and strengthens her body physically, especially her reproductive system.

Applications for Arousal: Before making love, have your partner lie down comfortably on her back with her eyes closed. Lightly touch this lower abdominal point. As you hold the point, encourage your partner to expand her belly with each inhalation. Ever so slowly increase your finger pressure at this point, while your other hand holds the lower back, strokes the breast and nipples, and then caresses the genital region. Stay on the Gate of Origin point for a while. You may begin to feel a pulsation there. This beneficial sign indicates that energy is flowing through the point. Continue to hold until the volume and speed of the pulse balances. Holding the point in this way often increases a woman's pleasure, no matter what sexual activity she then engages in, as long as she feels secure, trusting, and intimate.

AROUSAL ROUTINE FOR WOMEN

Before you begin, wash your partner's hands and feet with soap and water. Be sure your nails are short and filed smooth without any sharp edges; if your nails are long, be careful to use only the pads of your fingers. Stimulate each of the following arousal points for 1 or 2 minutes, spending longer on the areas your partner particularly enjoys.

Your partner is lying down on her back, with her legs comfortably spread apart.

1. Toe Suck (Sp 1, Lv 1). Give her a sensual foot massage using a nonscented vegetable oil such as almond oil. Massage her ankles, her heels, the bottoms and tops of her feet, and each toe. Sensually massage her feet, slowly gliding in between each toe. After you have covered the arches and balls of her feet, suck her toes. With your tongue, circulate around each toe before you suck it. Spend extra time sucking her large toes to stimulate Sp 1 and Lv 1. Lick and suck both large toes as you lightly caress her inner ankles with your fingertips.

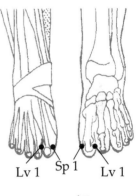

Top of Feet

2. Groin Press (Sp 12, Sp 13). Slide your fingertips slowly and gently up the insides of your partner's legs. Place the heels of your hands in the groin creases, where the thighs join the trunk of her body. Placing your fingertips lightly on her belly, slowly lean some of the weight of your chest into her groin points, gradually increasing the pressure toward her womb. You may feel a strong pulse underneath your palms. Adjust your hands comfortably, and hold for 2 minutes as you encourage her to breathe deeply into her belly.

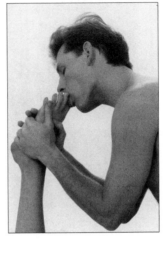

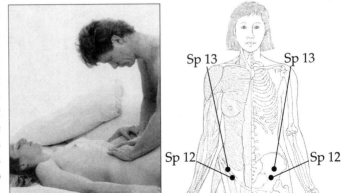

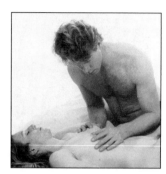

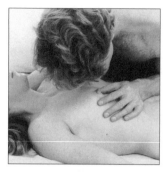

3. Nipple Roll (St 17). Glide your hands from your partner's groin upward along her sides to her nipples. Gently roll each nipple between your thumb and index finger. After a minute or two gradually increase the speed. Then kiss, lick, and firmly suck St 17 on one nipple as you roll the other nipple with your hand for at least a minute. Then suck the other side for another minute.

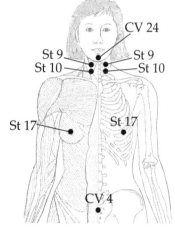

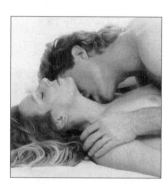

4. Neck Nibble (St 9, St 10). Gently kiss the points on her neck to further arouse her passions. You can stimulate these points even more by sucking them. At this point, you may feel like kissing passionately on the lips. Also try sucking CV 24, below the center of the lower lip for arousing a woman.

5. Sacral Press (B 27–B 34). Straddle her body, placing your hands underneath her to the base of her spine. Curve your fingers, using the weight of her body to press the sacral points.

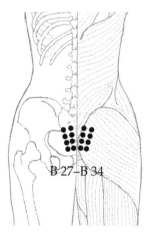

Sacral Points

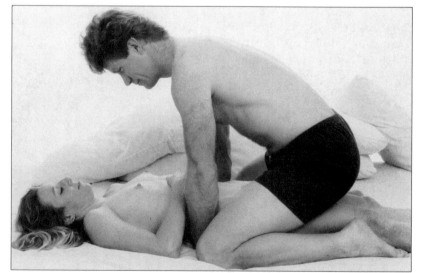

6. Connecting Vaginally with CV 4.
Slow deep pressure or sucking on the Gate of Origin (CV 4) can be especially arousing to a woman. As you place your palm over this point, use your other hand to lightly caress her thighs. Softly stroke upward, and tantalize her by fondling her anus and the hair between her legs. Gently touch the lips of her vagina with the pads of your fingers, using slow, circular movements, for at least 2 minutes. Enjoy feeling her moistness.

When she fully opens to you, gradually ease your index and middle fingers inside her. Use your fingertips to slowly glide over the roof of her vagina. With your fingers extended fully inside the vagina, slowly stroke the pads of your fingertips over the vaginal roof by curving your fingers. As you continue to repeat this finger movement, ask her for feedback to adjust your speed and pressure.

Glide slowly over the roof of her vagina in a circular motion as you palm her Gate of Origin. Being present and breathing deeply with her can be incredibly arousing.

7. Hold Her Sacral Points as You Touch Her Clitoris. Firmly press the base of her spine with the palm of one hand as you lightly touch her clitoris, between her vagina and her pubic bone, with the other hand. Gently hold the base of the clitoris with the pads of your fingertips, and verbally encourage her to breathe deeply into her belly and to move her pelvis against you. Enjoy being with each other; nothing is more important, sacred, loving, and precious.

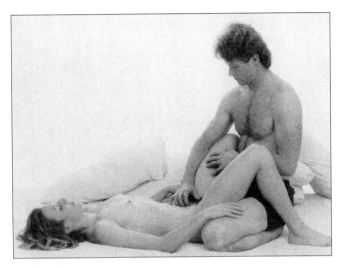

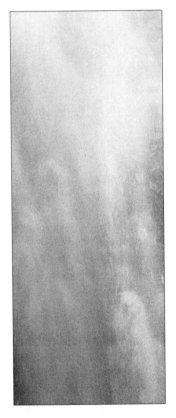

Chapter 7

AROUSING A MAN

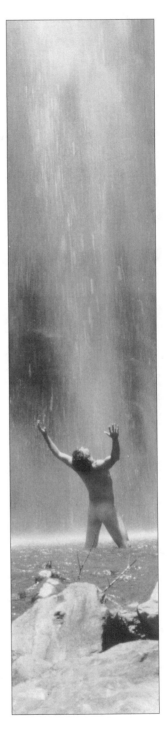

This chapter begins with an erotic practice for increasing a man's pleasure using acupressure, whether performed by a woman or another man. You will learn five sets of arousal points for men. All of these points are used in an acupressure Arousal Routine for Men at the end of the chapter.

INCREASING A MAN'S SEXUAL PLEASURE

Partners should first practice these techniques without the expectation of sexual excitement. Try them again at some other time for making love. To begin, the man lies on his back with his legs spread, his penis hanging downward. Kneel between his upper thighs.

1. **Place the heels of your hands on the creases where your partner's legs join the trunk of his body,** applying palm pressure. Let your fingers comfortably rest on his belly and place your thumbs over his pubic bone. Ask him to breathe slowly and deeply with you for a couple of minutes as you lean the weight of your chest over your hands. Encourage him to take long deep breaths into his belly, as if he were breathing into the pressure of your hands.

2. **Place your partner's penis on his lower abdominal area,** the head of it facing his navel. This works whether the penis is big or small, soft or hard. Men often enjoy having their penis pressed up against their belly. This upright position is similar to an erection, exposing the most vulnerable, sensitive side of the penis.

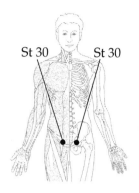

St 30   St 30

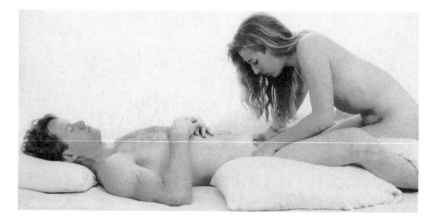

When a man learns

the techniques for

containing his ejacu-

lation, he is able to

make love for extended

periods of time. . . .

Longer periods of

lovemaking mean

more intimate sexual

play, more time for

communion through

intercourse, more of

those electric feelings of

arousal and desire and

supersensitivity and

pleasure.

—Charles and Caroline Muir
Tantra: The Art of Conscious Loving

Massage your partner's groin area. Then, rotate your fingers in toward each other, gradually placing your thumbs and index and middle fingers firmly over the penis. As you slowly lean your chest over your hands, the base of your thumbs and the heels of your hands will apply pressure to St 30, just beside the penis at the tip of the pubic bone. This point increases a man's genital sensitivity and thus heightens his sexual pleasure. When stimulating a man, be sure to include the testicles and scrotum. Most men love having their testicles caressed and felt.

Establish eye contact with your partner, expressing your intimate feelings and love through your gaze. Encourage him to breathe deeply into the pressure, as if he were breathing into his penis. The slower and deeper he breathes, the more feeling he will have. Invite your partner to slowly move his pelvis up and down, breathing deeply into the stimulation as you hold him.

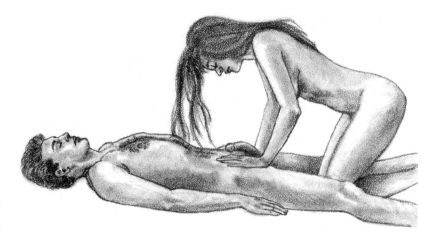

3. **Lightly stroke the hair surrounding his anus and scrotum.** Slowly caress him, starting from his anus up through the scrotum and the length of his penis. Barely touching the skin, tantalize every square inch between his legs while you continue to gaze into each other's eyes.

4. **Place the fingertips of one hand on the point midway between the anus and the scrotum (CV 1).** Rub in that area, and find a ropy cord there. Press firmly on that cord using your index, middle, and ring fingertips. Hold this point as the palm of your other hand rolls the penis from side to side over his pubic bone and belly. Gradually increase the speed of the rolling motion as your partner continues to breathe deeply into his belly.

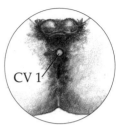

CV 1

5. **Slowly but firmly move your hand up and down the length of the penis,** creating friction on the exposed sensitive side. (You may wish to use a natural lubricant for additional pleasure.) As your partner breathes deeper and faster, increase the speed. Discovering the most erotic ways to treat your lover's main pleasure organ can be an exciting adventure.

6. **If you and your partner both desire to have intercourse,** slip his penis inside you. Place the heels of your hands above his pubic bone, and gradually lean some of your weight into his lower abdominal area, pressing the Sea of Intimacy points (CV 2–CV 6) to increase his sexual pleasure. Breathe deeply, and move in sync with him as you maintain eye contact and enjoy the warmth generated from your bodies.

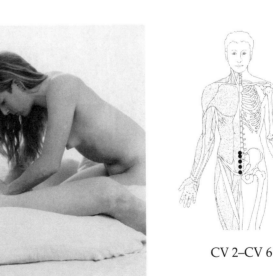

CV 2–CV 6

AROUSAL POINTS FOR MEN

You can incorporate any of these arousal points for men into the previous practice, Increasing a Man's Sexual Pleasure. You can also use these points by themselves as a simple way to begin an erotic journey with your partner. The arousal routine at the end of this section will instruct you how to use these points in a step-by-step sequence.

Sacral Points (B 27–B 34)

Pressing this series of points at the base of the spine properly can be quite arousing for a man. They are located in the small hollows of the plate of bone (sacrum) at the base of the spine. As you rub across this bone, feel for its small indentations. Pressing into these slight hollows triggers nerves that reach into the genitals. Holding these sacral points firmly for at least one minute can significantly increase sexual pleasure.

Some ancient peoples knew well the connection between the words *sacral* and *sacred*—sexuality was given the highest respect. When you and your partner press these Sacral Points to cultivate your full sexual life, you too may feel blessed, loved, and aroused and gain a sense of reverence.

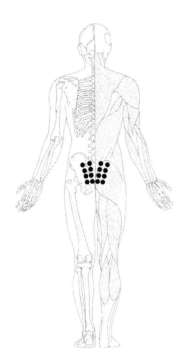

B 27–B 34

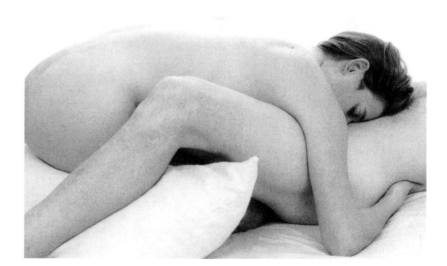

Sea of Intimacy (CV 2–CV 6)

The abdominal muscles often tighten during lovemaking. Since so many sexual sensations and movements commonly occur all at once, most people are unaware of this abdominal constriction. But left unattended, this tension can block your vital energy from flowing into your genitals and cause a wide range of sexual problems.

Pressing the acupressure points CV 2–CV 6 can effectively relieve abdominal tension, strengthen the urinary and reproductive systems, and increase sexual pleasure. Stimulating the Sea of Intimacy points twice a day (along with eating fish and avoiding products made with refined sugar) for at least 2 months can benefit a man who ejaculates prematurely. Couples who take a few minutes to press these points on each other in preparation for intercourse often find that their intimacy is enhanced.

Location: Two, three, four, five, and six finger-widths below the belly button. For people who are weak and sick, apply less pressure. Apply more pressure for people who are athletic and healthy. If the person has a medical condition, consult a qualified health professional with experience in acupressure. (He or she may recommend using a light touch.)

Applications for Arousal: Your partner is lying on his back. Sit close to his left side, and place your left hand under his lower back. Gradually squeeze the large ropy muscles on both sides, using your fingers and the heels of your hands. With your fingertips or the palm of your right hand, hold the Sea of Intimacy points as you encourage him to breathe deeply into his belly. If you apply the pressure gradually and he is generally healthy, you can go 1 to 2 inches deep into the abdomen. Hold these points for about 3 minutes as your partner continues deep belly breathing.

Gradually come off the lower back points, placing your left hand over your right hand in your partner's lower abdominal region. Slide your left hand down to his pubic bone, using the heel of your hand to press the acupressure points there. Hold this combination of points for another minute as your partner continues to breathe deeply.

Keeping your right hand on the Sea of Intimacy points, move your left hand off the pubic bone to CV 1, between the rectum and genitals. At this point between the legs, softly stroke the hairs of the scrotum up over the length of the penis several times, using a light touch.

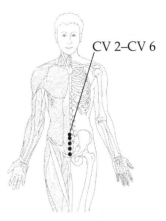

CV 2–CV 6

This region of the lower torso is the fountainhead of life-force which benefits health and longevity in general, and sexual vitality in particular.

—Valentin Chu
The Yin-Yang Butterfly

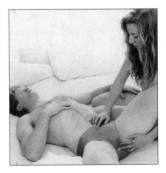

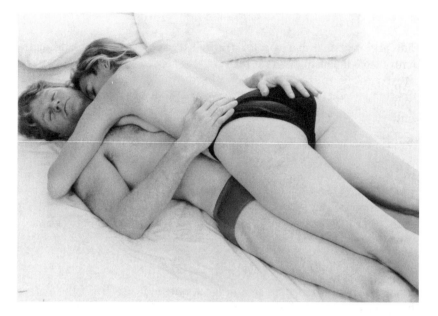

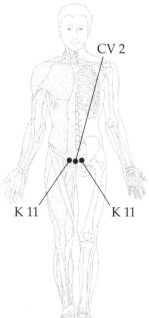

Crooked Bone (CV 2) *and Transverse Bone* (K 11)

Location: CV 2 is on the top edge of the pubic bone, in the center. K 11 is one-half finger-width from the midline, also on the upper edge (superior border) of the pubic bone.

Applications for Men: When you give your partner a full-body embrace while standing or lying down, explore the ways in which your pubic bones make contact. Depending upon each other's height, one partner may need to bend his or her knees or reach upward so that the pubic bones meet. When these bones are at the same level, gradually thrust your pelvis toward your partner until you feel the bones fit together and the pressure connects with your genitals.

Rushing Door and Mansion Cottage (Sp 12, Sp 13)

Location: Both points are in the pelvic area, in the middle of the crease where the leg joins the trunk of the body.

Applications for Men: Men often store their frustrations in these points. The tension that collects inhibits sexual energy from flowing into the genitals. It is important for a man to regularly release these points. He can learn how to press them himself. (See the Locust Pose in Chapter 3.) You can help him by following the instructions in Step 1 of Increasing a Man's Sexual Pleasure at the beginning of this chapter.

Inner Thigh (Lv 10–Lv 12)

Location: On the inside of the upper thigh, close to the inner crease where the thigh joins the trunk of the body.

Applications for Men: To arouse a man, try using a light touch to tantalize these points for a couple of minutes as a prelude to making love. Slowly and lightly stroke over Lv 10, Lv 11, and Lv 12 (in that order) several times to awaken a man's penis. Use your other hand to hold CV 1 between the genitals and the rectum. Gentle licks and kisses on these points can also be effective for arousing a man, especially before oral sex.

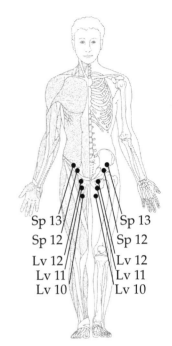

Sp 13 — Sp 13
Sp 12 — Sp 12
Lv 12 — Lv 12
Lv 11 — Lv 11
Lv 10 — Lv 10

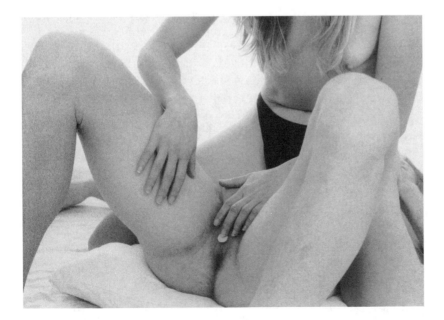

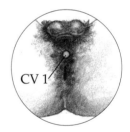

CV 1

AROUSAL ROUTINE FOR MEN

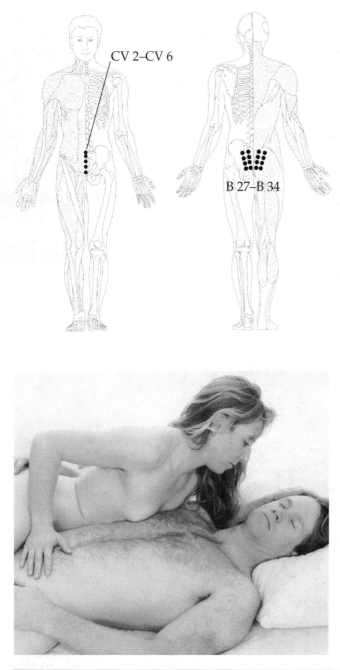

CV 2–CV 6

B 27–B 34

This routine is excellent to do before making love. Have your partner lie comfortably on his back. Take 5 minutes to relax him by slowly and firmly kneading his shoulders. Once his shoulder muscles feel more relaxed, use your thumbs, palms, or fists to press the large ropy muscles that run alongside his spine. Then continue with the following 5 sets of acupressure points. Stimulate each one for 1 to 2 minutes. Spend longer on the ones your partner particularly enjoys.

1. Sacral Press (B 27–B 34). With your fingertips or with the palms of your hands, apply pressure on the flat bone at the base of the spine (sacrum).

2. Lower Abdominal Press (CV 2–CV 6). Gradually apply pressure to these points using the pads of your fingertips on your partner's belly. Encourage him to breathe deeply while you continue to apply pressure. As he inhales, your hands will rise. As he exhales, let your hands slowly go deeper into his belly.

Ask your partner: "How's the pressure?" or "Would you like me to press a little higher or lower?" Continue holding and breathing deeply in sync with your partner for 2 or 3 minutes.

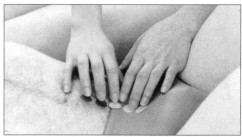

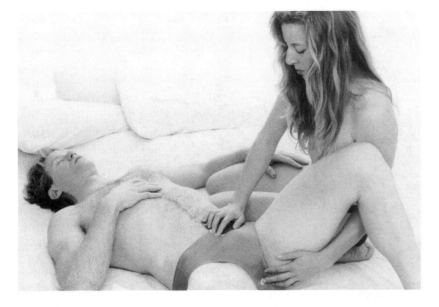

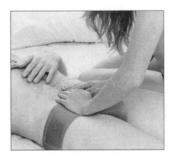

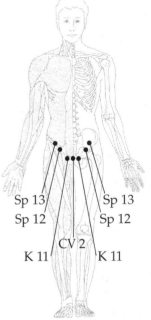

3. Pubic Sacral Press (CV 2, K 11). Place the heels of both your hands on the top of your partner's pubic bone. Your fingers rest on top of his belly. Ask him to explore making erotic movements with his pelvis. Both you and your partner should breathe deeply into your bellies as you hold these points for a couple of minutes.

4. Groin Press (Sp 12, Sp 13). Place the heels of your hands on the groin creases where the thighs join the trunk of the body. Position the base of your thumbs so that they are touching the outside tips of your partner's pubic bone. With your fingertips lightly on his belly, slowly lean the weight of your chest over his groin points, gradually increasing the pressure. Encourage him to breathe into his belly. You should feel a strong pulse. Adjust your hands for your comfort, and hold for 2 minutes while breathing deeply.

Sp 13   Sp 13
Sp 12   Sp 12
CV 2
K 11   K 11

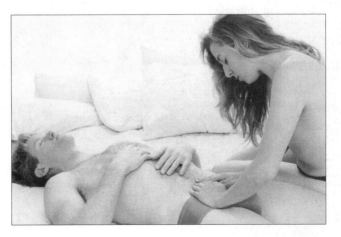

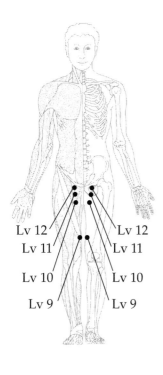

Lv 12   Lv 12
Lv 11   Lv 11

Lv 10   Lv 10

Lv 9   Lv 9

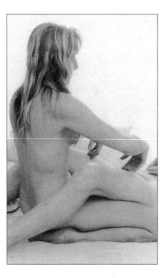

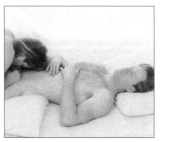

5. Thigh Fondle (Lv 9–Lv 12). Gently glide your fingertips up your partner's inner thighs, starting at Lv 9. Lightly stroke up to Lv 12. Continue to caress his inner thighs, each time coming a little bit closer to his genitals as you both maintain eye contact.

Reposition your partner's legs with his knees bent and comfortably spread outward, and his feet flat on the floor. Breathe deeply as you gently caress his inner thighs up to CV 1. Place his penis over the pubic bone onto his belly. Continue to stroke his thighs, starting at Lv 9. Now very slowly glide up his thighs, through the scrotum, to the tip of his penis.

Once he is fully aroused and erect, lower yourself onto him and firmly rub the warmth of your belly against his penis. Breathe deeply as you reach out your feet to connect with his. Enjoy moving against each other and breathing deeply together in celebration of your erotic full-body contact.

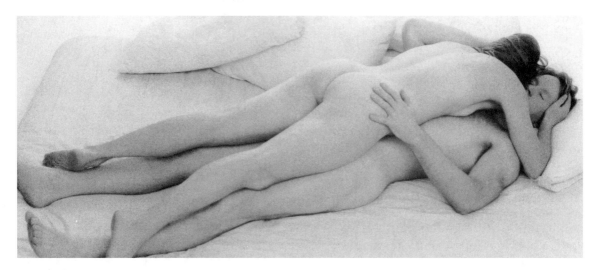

Chapter 8

ACUPRESSURE FOR MUTUAL STIMULATION

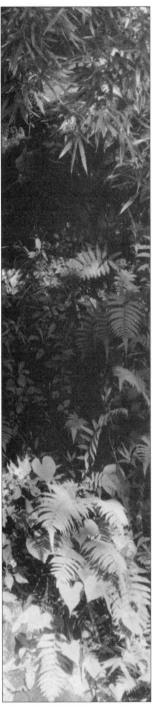

*T*his chapter tells you about routines and points that are sexually stimulating and that can be used for sensual arousal, mutual gratification, or as a prelude to other sexual activities.

MUTUAL FOOT MASSAGE

Reflexology, the healing art of hand and foot massage, is based upon the fact that thousands of nerves end in the hands and on the soles of the feet. Thoroughly massaging the hands and feet stimulates these nerve endings, sending benefits to every area of the body.

Try giving your partner this luxurious foot massage after a long day at work, whether for rejuvenation or as prelude to making love. You can also try this massage to unwind before going to sleep.

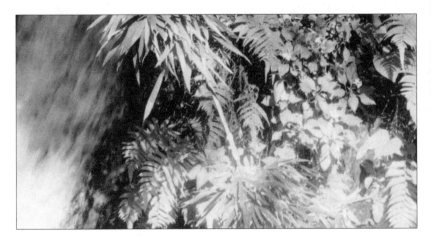

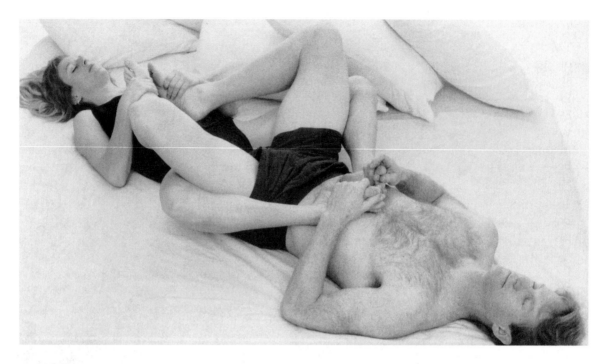

1. Have your partner lie down on his or her back, feet spread wide apart. Place your buttocks in between your partner's thighs, and lie down on your back, with the top of your head pointing in the opposite direction from your partner's.

2. Both of you bend your knees, gently placing your feet onto each other's abdomen, with the soles comfortably apart. If you find this awkward, adjust the distance between your buttocks as well as the positioning of your feet until you both find a comfortable position.

3. Slowly massage your partner's feet: firmly grasp, knead, and caress them. Be sure to cover the bottoms of the feet, the arches, ankles, and toes.

Suggestions

- The less limber partner should have his or her feet on top of the other's legs. The partner on top provides a weight for gently stretching the inner thighs of the partner below. The more your partner's legs relax outward, the more weight will be applied to gently stretch your legs.

- Whenever the person whose legs are underneath finds it to be too much of a stretch, simply switch. When the lighter partner is on the bottom, be especially careful not to apply too much pressure to the stretch.

- To relieve tightness on the insides of your thighs, have your partner position his or her heels in the inner groin just beside your genitals, gradually applying pressure to the tight muscles in this area. Meanwhile, change your position by simply lifting your heels up, placing them in the hollows on either side of your lover's pubic bone. Gradually applying firm pressure in this area helps to release the abductor muscles, which in Eastern sexology are connected with the sexual-reproductive system.

You are my likeness, for we are prisoners of two bodies formed of one clay. You are my companion on the road of life and my helper in the understanding of a truth concealed beyond the clouds.

—Kahlil Gibran
A Tear and a Smile

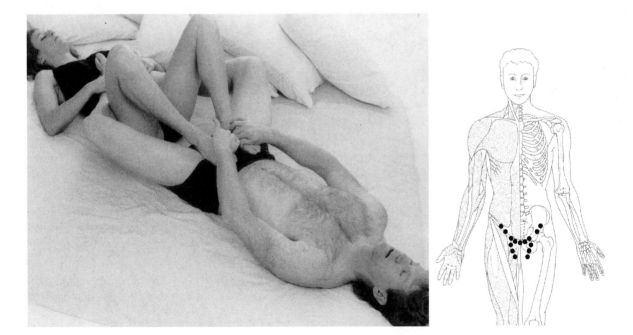

117

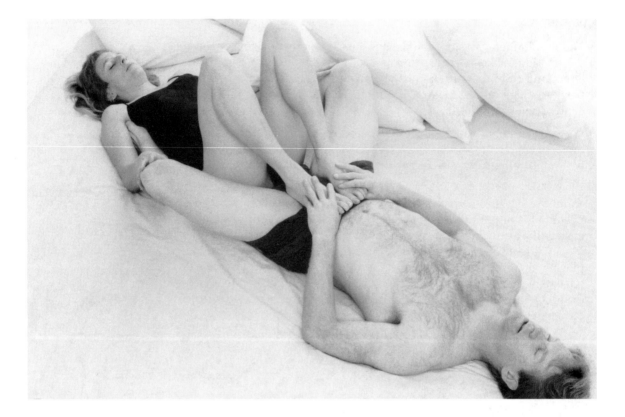

Variations

- You can place your feet in various positions for this mutual foot massage. Instead of putting both feet on the abdomen, you can bend your knees and place your feet flat on the floor beside your partner's hips. Meanwhile, your partner places his or her feet in your groin, on or just beside the pubic bone.

- With your legs bent and the bottoms of the feet together, place the sides of your feet on the center of your partner's chest. Your partner can place his or her heels in the crease where your thigh joins your genital region.

- With the soles of your partner's feet on the top of your pubic bone, place your heels in your partner's armpits with his or her arms extended outward.

• With your partner's knees bent toward his or her chest, place your feet on the outside of the shinbone, three inches beneath the knee, on St 36. Slowly arch your pelvis upward as you push your feet against your lover's legs, bringing the knees closer to the chest.

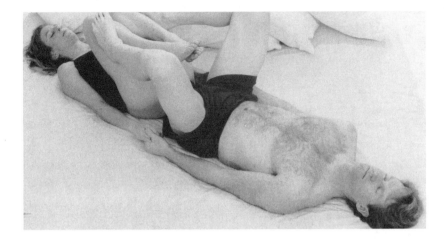

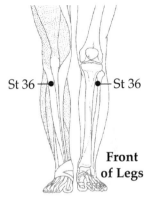

St 36 — St 36

Front of Legs

• Place your feet in the back of your partner's thighs, with your heels on points B 50 and B 51. The soles of your partner's feet remain on St 36. Slowly arch your pelvis upward, and gently push your feet against your partner's thighs, applying firm pressure. Then relax down. By doing this rhythmically, you can create a rocking motion.

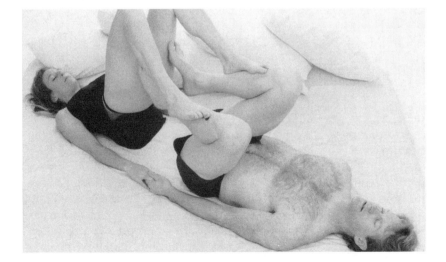

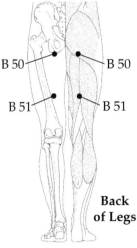

B 50 — B 50

B 51 — B 51

Back of Legs

Once you switch roles giving and receiving, scoot closer. This time, try interlacing your fingers for an even greater connection.

ACUPRESSURE POINTS

K 1–K 6 are stimulated in the Mutual Foot Massage.

The Sp, K, and Lv meridians are stretched in this posture.

CV 2–CV 17 are stimulated by the sides of the feet.

Lv 3, St 44, and GB 41, on the tops of the feet, are stimulated with the thumbs in the foot massage.

B 53–B 54 are stimulated on the backs of the knees.

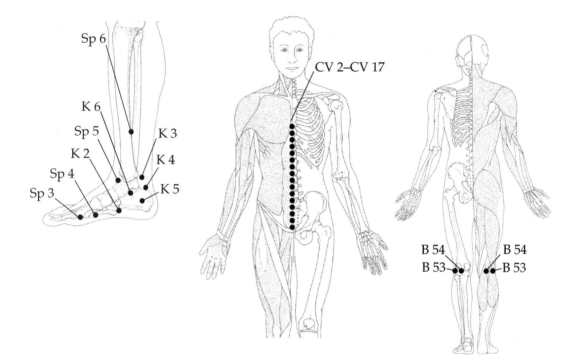

Benefits: The Mutual Foot Massage stimulates the reflexology points corresponding to all organs and parts of the body. In addition, the postures and movements gently stretch the spleen, kidney, and liver meridians. Putting the bottoms of your feet against the back of your partner's thighs and calves stimulates the bladder meridian. Placing the sides of your feet on your partner's lower abdominal area and groin stimulates the liver, spleen, stomach, and kidney meridians as well as Conception Vessel points. In addition, propping your head up with a couple of pillows enables you to talk intimately with your partner and make eye contact while touching each other.

SENSUAL INTIMACY

The more awake your senses are, the greater your capacity for intimacy and love. Sadly, Western culture tends to be sensually limiting. When it comes to making love, we often deny our sensual needs, deodorize our bodies, numb ourselves with drugs, and darken the room. Yet to honor your partner with your full attention and to deepen your relationship, you need all of your senses.

Just as a parent delights in the wondrous smells of a baby, a man can appreciate a woman's natural perfumes: the cyclical shifts in her bodily fragrances and the bouquet of her sexual juices. A woman can enjoy the rich scents of a man's hair, his sweat, and muskiness.

As you make love, notice the expressions in your partner's face, the movements of greeting, appreciation, and love. Savor each experience, each sexual exchange you share. Delight in the feel and texture of your partner's body; explore its shapes and openings.

As you open all your senses, be conscious of giving to your partner with all your heart. Breathe deeply. Remember that the love and attention you give returns to you, strengthening your relationship.

When all of your body's senses are awakened, your intimacy increases. Sharing sensual pleasure exposes yourself, showing your partner what you deeply feel and enjoy as well as what enlivens you.

I believe in the flesh and the appetites. Seeing, hearing, and feeling are miracles, and each part and tag of me is a miracle.

—Walt Whitman
Leaves of Grass

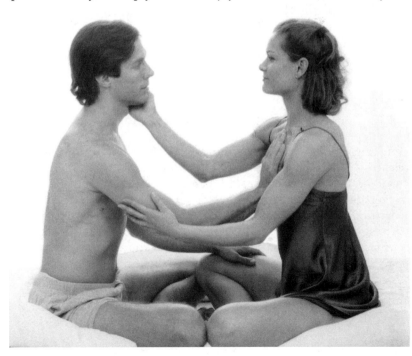

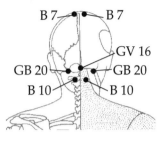

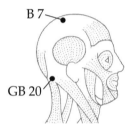

The point of love is not to pin it down or provide a formula for being so that the rational self can feel safe and secure. The point of love is to invite us to reach deeper into our experience.

—Richard Moss, M.D.
The I That Is We

FOUR GATES FOR REAWAKENING SENSUAL SENSITIVITY

Acupressure can heighten your sensuality because each acupressure point is a sensory gateway. When your points are blocked, your senses are not clear, inhibiting your ability to perceive your own feelings, interpret your body's messages, and receive information about the world around you, including from your partner.

These four primary points are major gateways for enhancing your sensuality. Experiment with them on each other's bodies, to see which are most beneficial to you. Hold the most responsive points for 2 to 3 minutes each, and spend about a minute on the others. Follow this point sequence:

1. *Heavenly Pillar* (B 10). These important neurological points on the back of the neck enhance sensual awareness.
2. *Penetrating Heaven* (B 7). Located on the top of the head, these points open your sense of smell as well as your intuition.
3. *Wind Mansion* (GV 16). Located in the large hollow in the center underneath the base of your skull, this point relaxes and quiets your mind and central nervous system, enabling you to have greater awareness of your senses.
4. *Gates of Consciousness* (GB 20). At the base of the skull lie these primary points for heightening intimate experiences and increasing sensory awareness.

TEN SENSUAL INTIMACY POINTS

Touching can be both sensual and intimate when you are deeply relaxed with your partner. Where and how you touch each other can create erotic feelings. Intimate touch is like fire—it requires ample oxygen. Slow deep breathing is essential for fueling sensual intimacy when you touch each other's most pleasurable erotic areas.

These ten following acupressure points are located in highly sensual parts of the body. They can open a romantic, erotic way of being. Remember to breathe deeply together and touch each other slowly while using them. The Sensual Intimacy Routine at the end of this section suggests how to use these arousing points in a step-by-step sequence.

Heavenly Pond (P 1)

Location: One thumb-width outside the nipple.

Benefits: Holding this point nurtures the spirit in the heart, increases sexual intimacy, and cultivates the expression of love.

Applications for Sensuality:

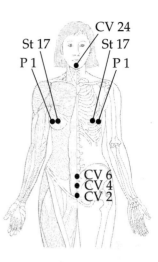

- Caress this lovely point for increasing intimacy toward the end of a nurturing massage or before making love.

- Lightly touch or hold this point to nourish your partner. Another name for this sensitive point is Heaven's Pool, which refers to gathering love into our breasts and nurturing the "pillows of our hearts." After a man gently touches P 1 on his partner, he can enjoy sucking the St 17 point on her nipple while breathing deeply.

- Before making love, explore P 1 with gentle kisses and licks, as well as St 17 on the nipples, while you touch CV 24, below the center of the lower lip. As you continue to nurture Heavenly Pond, slowly glide your hand down to hold CV 6, CV 4, and CV 2, in that order. After enjoying love-play and caresses, lightly explore your lover's favorite pleasurable terrains.

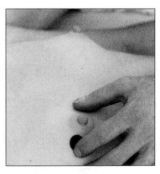

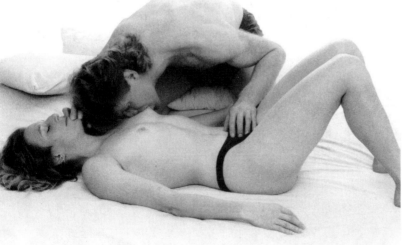

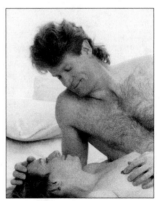

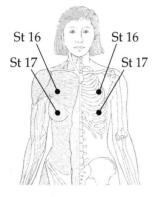

St 16   St 16
St 17   St 17

Breast Window (St 16) and Center of the Breasts (St 17)

Location: St 16 is above the breast tissue, just inside of the nipple line, between the third and fourth ribs. St 17 is in the center of the nipple.

Benefits: Increases emotional vulnerability, compassion, and an intimate spirit.

Applications for Sensuality:

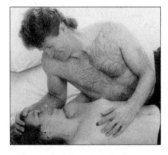

- Gently hold each of these points with your fingertips as your other hand firmly supports the area directly in back between your partner's shoulder blades. Holding the front and back of the body in this way cultivates emotional intimacy and openness.

- As you hold Breast Window (St 16), affectionately caress your lover's face, head, and hair, while looking into his or her eyes.

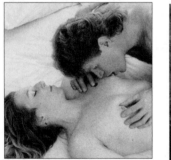

- Breast Window is also an excellent point to hold while you suck on your partner's nipple, which stimulates St 17.

- Caress these points for enhancing intimacy during a nurturing massage or before making love.

- For arousing a woman using St 17, see Chapter 6. A Loving Lounge Chair in Chapter 10 explains how to use this point in preparation for intercourse.

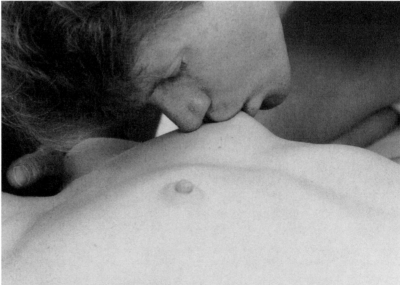

Rushing Door (Sp 12) *and Mansion Cottage* (Sp 13)

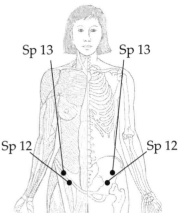

These two points are especially effective for increasing sexual intimacy and lessening menstrual discomfort.

Location: In the pelvic area, in the middle of the crease where the leg joins the trunk of the body.

Benefits: Touching these points particularly enhances sensations in the genitals.

Applications for Sensuality:

- With your partner lying on his or her back, gently place the heel of your hands on the groin crease. Slowly lean into the Rushing Door points with the heels of your hands. If you feel a strong throbbing pulsation in the groin, hold the points a few minutes longer until the throbbing evens out. Then cuddle close to your partner, embracing him or her affectionately.

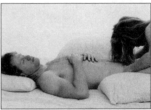

- For other applications using these points, see Touching the Delights Below, later in this chapter.

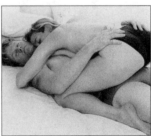

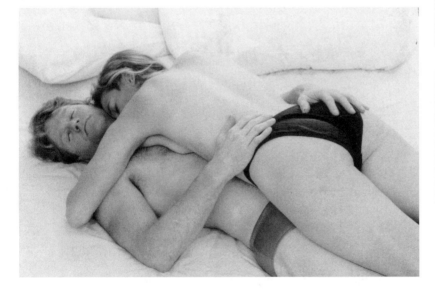

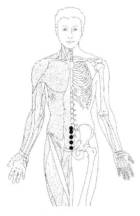

CV 2–CV 6

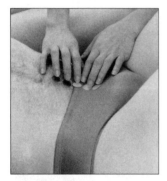

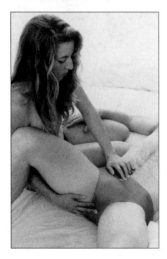

Sea of Intimacy (CV 2–CV 6)

Caution: Apply less pressure to people who are weak or sick, more pressure to those who are athletic and healthy. If a person has a medical condition, disease, or weakness, consult a qualified health professional with experience in acupressure, and use a light touch.

Location: Between two and seven finger-widths below the navel.

Benefits: Touching these points restores, secures, and supplements sexual intimacy.

Applications for Sensuality:

- Place the fingertips of one hand on CV 6, an inch and a half below the navel. Very gradually increase the pressure, taking one full minute to descend slowly one inch into the abdomen. As you breathe slowly and deeply in sync with your partner, use your other hand to sensually touch CV 1, between the rectum and genitals. Continue to breathe deeply together.

- For other applications using these points, see Touching the Delights Below, later in this chapter, as well as the intercourse positions in Chapter 10.

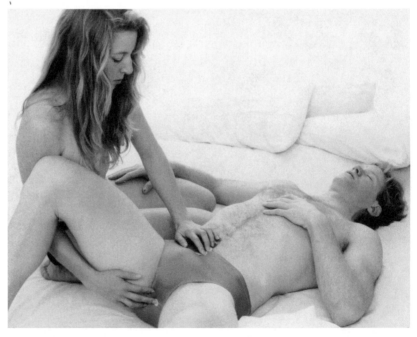

Supporting Nourishment (CV 24)

Location: In the indentation midway between the center of the lower lip and chin.

Benefits: Touching this point relaxes the facial muscles. Touching it in a romantic setting increases intimacy and erotic feelings through enhancing awareness of your lips and your sexual energy.

Applications for Sensuality:

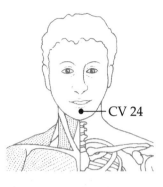

- Lightly touching this point while your bodies are close together in a private, comfortable environment often creates an intimate connection. Erotic intimacy may build if you open your partner's lips while touching this point, breathing deeply together and gazing intensely into each other's eyes.

- Touching and kissing this point can deepen a sexual experience. When you are on top of your partner engaging in intercourse, try sucking this point. Communicate how much you want your partner by the intensity of the suction. You can also stimulate this sensual intimacy point without having intercourse. Sometime when you are passionately kissing in bed, explore how it feels to have this point sucked erotically.

- You will find other applications for using this point in Enjoying Each Other's Bodies, later in this chapter, and in Embracing Love and A Reconnecting Couple's Routine in Chapter 9.

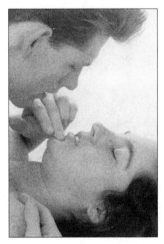

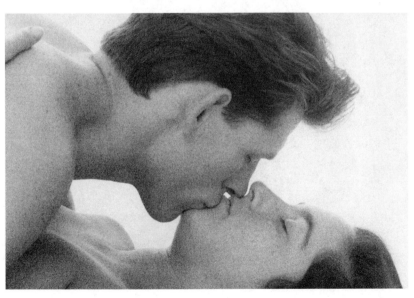

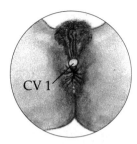

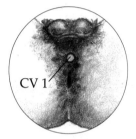

Inner Meeting (CV 1)

Location: At the center of the perineum, midway between the anus and genitals.

Benefits: Touching this intimate point enhances orgasm and benefits the reproductive organs. In addition, it relieves pressure in the genitals and rectum, impotence and premature ejaculation.

Applications for Sensuality:

• Encourage your partner to breathe deeply as you hold CV 1 between the anus and genitals. With your other hand, gently caress the palms, the insides of your partner's arms and breasts, and the area around the ears. Be sure to touch your partner on both sides.

• Your partner lies on his or her back with knees bent outward. Hold CV 1 with one hand as you sensitively touch his or her feet, inner ankles, calves, and inner thighs with your other hand. Take your time to tantalize the genitals.

• CV 1 is an invaluable acupressure point for lovers. After a bath or shower, an adventurous couple may enjoy exploring different ways to stimulate it with the tip of the tongue or gentle kisses.

• For using this acupressure point in different postures, see Erotic Oral Sex in Chapter 9 and A Loving Lounge Chair in Chapter 10.

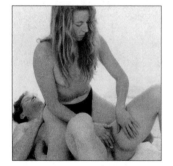

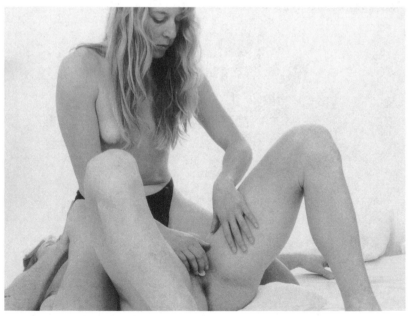

SENSUAL INTIMACY ROUTINE

Throughout these steps, your partner lies comfortably on his or her back and breathes slowly and deeply. Sit by the waist, facing your partner's head.

1. Gently stroke the palms, inner arms, neck, and ears. Encourage your partner to breathe into the sensual pleasures of your touch.

2. Lightly caress the breasts (P 1, St 16, St 17). Gently and slowly, tantalize your partner's breasts with your palms and fingertips as you make eye contact and breathe deeply together.

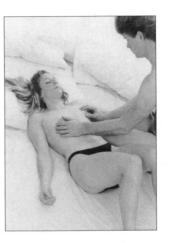

3. Palm the groin and lower belly (Sp 12, Sp 13, CV 2–CV 6). Gradually place your palms in the groin on Sp 12 and Sp 13, and turn your hands to place your fingertips on CV 2, CV 3, CV 4, CV 5, and CV 6. Now deepen your breathing and continue to explore each other through gazing into each other's eyes.

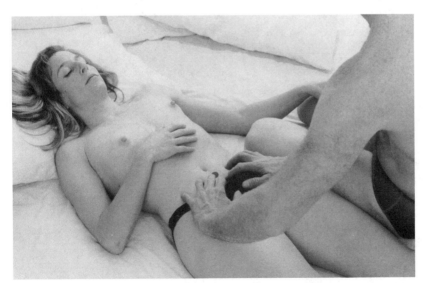

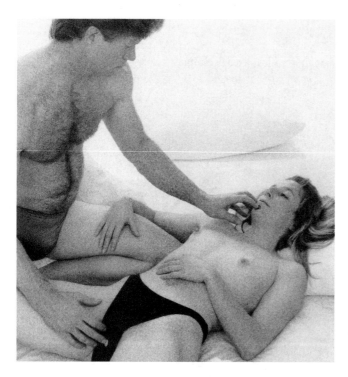

4. Touch above and below (CV 24 and CV 1). With one hand, hold the point between your partner's chin and lower lip, while your other hand searches for the point between the anus and genitals. Continue your eye gazing and breathing together in sync.

5. Give a full-body embrace. (This gets all the points!) Then slowly move closer together. Savor the moment before you hug. As you begin to embrace, gently slide over each other's body until you feel your bones fit together with your partner's like puzzle pieces. Once you feel your bodies completely connect from head (your temples together) to toe (your feet or ankles touching), wrap your arms as far around your partner as you can. Reach and gradually pull your beloved into your heart, breathing deeply together as one.

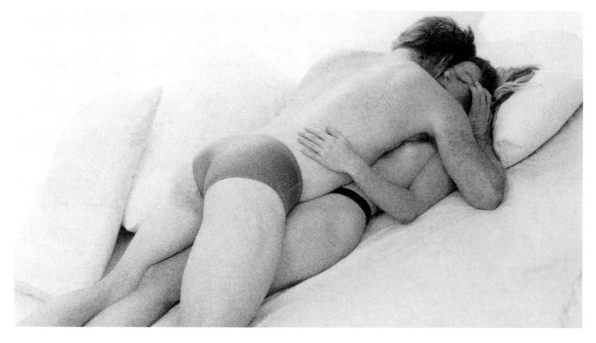

EXPLORING NEW POSTURES

Most couples tend to repeat the same familiar sexual activities, and after a while these motions can lose their excitement. Thus it is vital to explore new strokes, postures, and activities, provided you are both open to expanding your repertoire. The following couple's exercises encourage you to explore new ways of touching each other.

When they first try these postures, most couples find it easier to leave their clothes on. At this stage, nudity may distract you from experiencing new ways of bringing your bodies together.

Explore these postures in different environments. Try practicing them not only on your bed but on a bedsheet placed on a carpeted floor. Couples who work out regularly tend to prefer firmer surfaces; those with softer or more sensitive bodies often prefer their bed. It's always helpful to have pillows nearby for props.

Each of us has different preferences for how we like to be held and touched. For instance, it is important for you and your partner to discover who is more comfortable on the bottom and who on top. Try both positions, sharing verbally what works best. One of you may find certain new postures awkward. Feel free to skip the exercises that don't work well, or make the necessary adjustments.

In each posture, try various movements. Slowly rock your pelvis. Subtly move your head in rhythm with your breathing: As your head comes upward, inhale; as it comes downward, exhale. Hold, touch, or massage different areas of your partner's body. Again, communicate your preferences and body awarenesses with your partner, for openness is a key to intimacy.

To get the most enjoyment out of the exercises and to enable your bodies to adjust, be sure to move slowly—the slower, the better. Your touch will be far more powerful if you move your hands slowly. Also move slowly during the transitions between each posture. Hurried movements can break the mood.

If they let themselves come gradually into contact, they create a situation in which their senses can really work, so that when they have discovered what it can mean just to touch hands, the intimacy of a kiss or even lips in near proximity regains the electric quality which it had at the first meeting. . . . Intimacy just leads to passion.

—Alan Watts
Sex as a Contemplative Activity

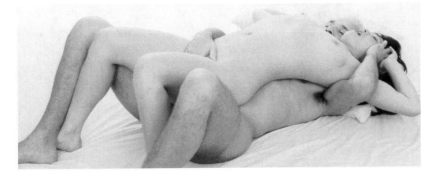

131

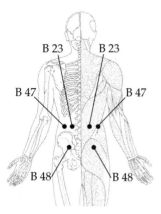

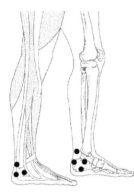

Riding Your Lover

Directions

1. Sit on the floor with your legs straight out in front. (If your partner is larger than you are, he or she should sit on the floor.)

2. Facing your feet, your partner straddles your legs in a kneeling position, being careful not to put all of his or her weight on your legs. This is a good position for mutual massage.

3. Your partner grasps the many points around your ankles and massages your feet from this kneeling position.

4. Lean forward and massage your partner's lower back and buttocks, to stimulate points B 23, B 47, and B 48.

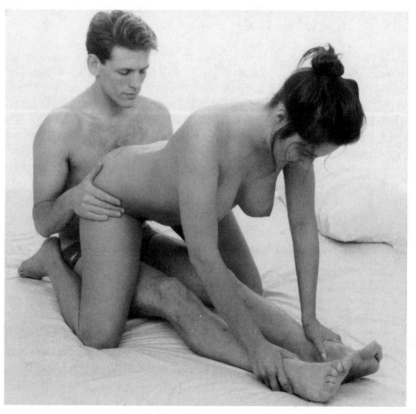

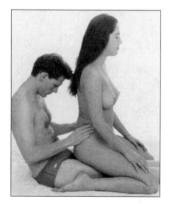

Advanced Variations

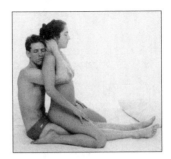

- Your partner moves back, straddling your legs near your lap in a squatting position. Bring your arms underneath your partner's armpits into a full nelson. With the heel of your hands, press and massage your partner's neck as you slowly stretch him or her forward and gently downward.

- Wrap your arms around your partner's waist. As you hug, slowly lean backward, lying down on your back with your lover on top of you. Adjust your heads comfortably side by side.

- As your partner lies down on top of you, align the base of his or her spine (the sacrum) on top of your pubic bone, stimulating points St 30, K 11, and CV 2. Adjust your bodies so they fit together comfortably to connect with these sacral points (B 27–B 34) at the base of the spine.

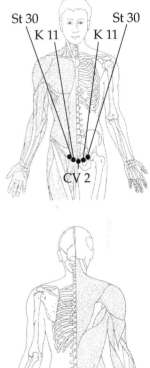

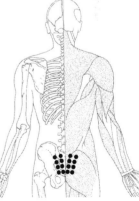

B 27–B 34

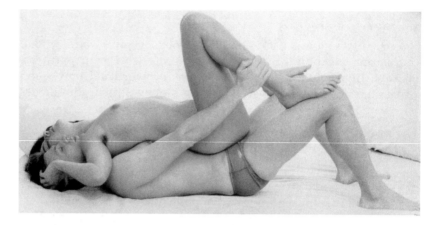

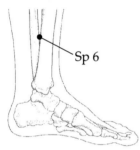

Sp 6

- Spread your legs outward. Your partner places his or her feet inside with knees bent. Then bend your knees, bringing your feet up onto your lover's thighs. Your partner grasps your lower shins, pulling them up to his or her groin.

- Both partners wrap their fingers around the outside of each other's leg, to the Three Yin Meeting point (Sp 6) approximately 4 finger-widths above the inner ankle bone. Breathe slowly and deeply together as your pelvises thrust in unison.

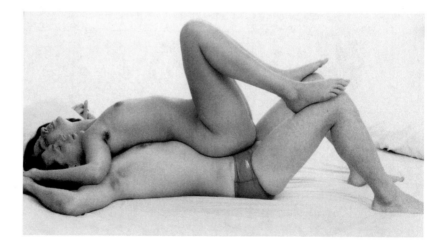

Spooning

Cuddle with your partner, without any expectations. Move your bodies together until you feel close to each other, heart to heart, talking intimately about your lives. Find a comfortable way to hold each other as you share your day, your thoughts, your appreciation, and concerns.

Directions

1. Lie on your sides, with your heads about a foot apart on pillows in a semifetal position. Comfortably spoon your partner from behind, extending your bottom arm under his or her neck. Breathe slowly and deeply together, relaxing and synchronizing your breath.
2. Your partner bends his or her upper leg, bringing the foot flat on the floor. Bring your upper leg over your partner's thigh.
3. Your bottom leg rests on the floor, straight out. Your partner's bottom leg bends until the bottom of that foot rests on top of your foot.
4. Gracefully bring your upper arm to the top of your partner's head, fitting the heel of the hand onto his or her temple. Massage your partner's scalp; breathe deeply together.

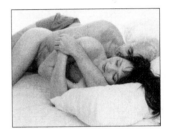

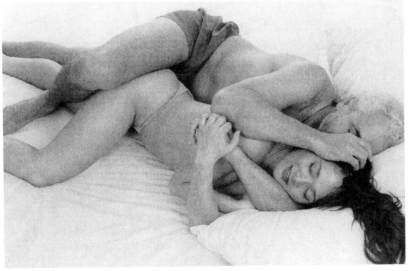

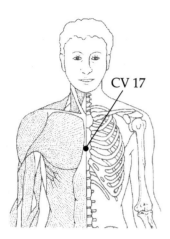

CV 17

Variations

- Lying on your side, slowly scoot back a few inches, rolling your partner onto his or her back. The knee of your partner's upper leg gradually comes up toward you, straddling your waist.

- Bend your top leg upward, placing it between your partner's legs. Readjust your body to rest your knee gently on your partner's groin or thigh.

- Place the palm of your upper hand on the center of your partner's breastbone (CV 17) as he or she comfortably places his or her hands on your body. Breathe deeply together.

Suggestions

- With your legs bent slightly more, cuddle a little closer, fitting your bodies together like puzzle pieces.

- Turning your heads toward each other, gaze into each other's eyes as you breathe deeply together.

- Try different ways to hold hands in this position while you talk, touch, or lovingly play together.

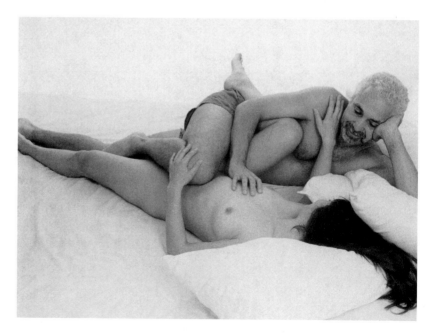

Acupressure Points

Point	Name	Location
CV 17	*Sea of Tranquility*	On the center of the breastbone, four finger-widths up from the base of the breastbone
Sp 10	*Sea of Blood*	Three finger-widths above the kneecap on the inside of the thigh
Sp 12 Sp 13	*Rushing Door* *Mansion Cottage*	In the groin, on the crease where the thigh meets the trunk of the body
GB 21	*Shoulder Well*	On the highest point of the top of the shoulder muscle, one to two inches from the side of the lower neck
Sp 6	*Three Yin Meeting*	Four finger-widths above the inner ankle bone
Sp 4	*Grandparent-Grandchild*	On the arch of the foot one thumb-width away from the ball of the foot
Lv 10 Lv 11	*Inward Pleasure*	On the top of the inner thigh, close to the genitals
Lv 9	*Joy of Living*	One-third of the way up from the knee toward the inner groin, on the inside of the thigh between the muscles

Benefits: Pressing the spleen, liver, and gallbladder points in these postures relieves frustrations and replenishes both the female and male reproductive organs.

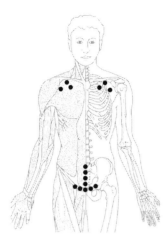

Riding the Sea of Intimacy

When your bodies fully embrace and fit together, they naturally stimulate key acupressure points. This direct contact enables your vital energy systems to connect, like jumper cables in a car.

The energy current created while making love, playing together, or simply hugging is not only intensely pleasurable but can activate healing energies and circulate energy throughout the body. This couple's exercise uses your body as a tool to relieve tensions and heal. It uses the whole body to stimulate points in the pelvic region, all of which, including the Sea of Intimacy, increase sexual depth and overall vitality.

Note: Do not do this exercise if your partner has a life-threatening disease or health condition.

Directions: Your partner lies on his or her back, a pillow under the head, knees bent, feet flat on the floor. Straddle the midsection of your partner's body facing his or her head. Slowly lower yourself down, and sit on your partner's pubic bone. Massage your partner's chest area, while he or she massages your knees and legs.

It is the love of the adventure and tremendous intimacy of sharing and receiving at the very boundaries of our being that enlivens me. It is passionate. It is sensuous in ways I could have never imagined.

—Richard Moss, M.D.
The I That Is We

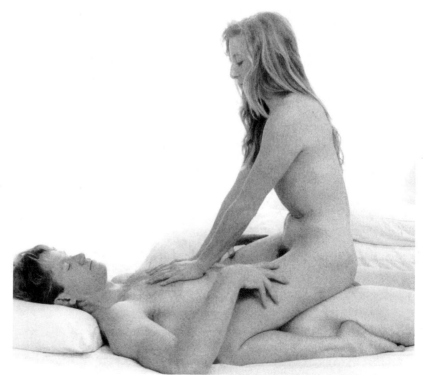

Suggestions

- Slowly rock your upper body backward and forward, constantly shifting your body's weight distribution.

- Slowly slide your buttocks onto your partner's *hara* (the vital center located midway between the navel and the pubic bone).

Variations

Your partner keeps his or her legs together and bent for these variations.

- Interlace your fingers firmly together, gazing into each other's eyes. Lean toward your partner, sustaining eye contact. Breathe slowly and deeply together.

- Slowly lean back onto your partner's thighs, and bring your arms over your head. Breathe and relax, enjoying the upper back stretch.

- Bring your arms down and massage your partner's buttocks. Make slow pelvic movements together as you take long, slow deep breaths. Firmly knead your partner's buttock muscles, while he or she grasps your hips and massages your groin with the thumbs. The pubic and genital areas can also be explored.

- Bring your upper body forward in a straddling position. Interlace your fingers with your partner's. Gaze deeply into each other's eyes, or kiss passionately. Continue to breathe deeply together. Enjoy the intimate connection of being present in the moment with each breath, sigh, glance, smile, and movement.

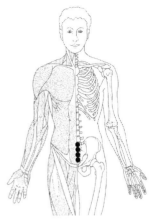

Points in the Hara

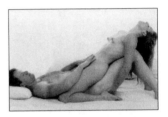

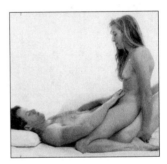

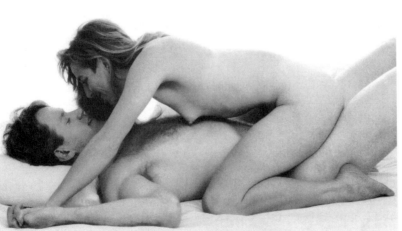

Acupressure Points

Point	Name	Location
GB 21	*Shoulder Well*	On the highest point of the top of the shoulder muscle, one to two inches from the side of the lower neck
Lu 1	*Letting Go*	On the outer part of the chest, three finger-widths below the collarbone
Sp 19	*Chest Village*	On the outer part of the chest, five and six finger-widths below the collarbone
Sp 20	*Encircling Glory*	
K 11	*Transverse Bone*	One half-inch from the midline of the pubic bone
K 12	*Great Brightness*	One finger-width above K 11
K 13	*Energy Hole*	Two finger-widths above K 11
K 14	*Four Full*	Three finger-widths above K 11
CV 2–CV 6	*Sea of Intimacy*	In the center of the lower abdomen, between the navel and the pubic bone
St 27	*Great Night*	In a direct line up from the edge of the pubic bone (St 30)
St 28	*Water Path*	
St 29	*The Return*	
St 30	*Energy Rushing*	Three finger-widths out from the center of the pubic bone, at the outer tips of this bone

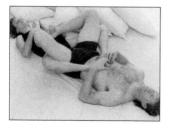

Going Further: From this position, your partner can drop his or her knees outward, spreading his or her legs open. You slide backward and sit on the floor between your partner's knees. Lie back on the floor, placing the bottoms of your feet together on your partner's abdomen. This couple's position easily leads to the Mutual Foot Massage described earlier in this chapter.

Enjoying Each Other's Bodies

The next exercise naturally enables couples to be close and intimate. You may need to reread the directions a few times and patiently try various positions before you discover how to fit together in this comfortable full-body intertwine. Once you find it, you will be in an excellent position for passionate kissing, talking, and beginning to make love.

Enjoying Each Other's Bodies is a sacred way to attune and communicate, not only through words but through eye contact and touch. Stay fully present with your partner to experience the depths of your intimacy in this romantic intertwine.

Directions

1. Your partner lies on his or her back, with a pillow underneath his or her head.
2. Lie down facing your partner on your side in a semifetal position, with your head propped up on a hand.
3. Your partner brings the leg that is closest to your body up and over your waist, placing his or her buttocks snug against your stomach. Your partner's other leg slides in between your legs. Reposition your legs until they feel comfortable and seem to fit together.

She rubbed my back and my side and finally my rear end. She unbuttoned my shirt as her lips moved slowly down my neck. She stripped me down and I did the same to her. We made passionate love like in the movies. That moment was so intense I'll never forget it.

—Jack Morin
The Four Cornerstones of Eroticism

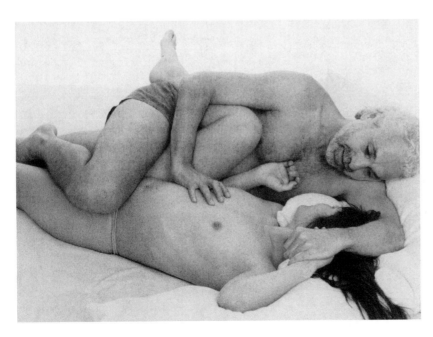

Suggestions

- Gently caress each other's face, and gaze into each other's eyes. Try touching your partner's forehead, or knead his or her shoulders.

- Gently massage the leg draped over your waist, ending with several light, silky, tantalizing strokes.

Variation: Romantic Intertwine

1. Snuggle close, positioning yourself up high on your forearm and elbow. Bend your upper leg, placing the top of your thigh against your partner's genitals. Maintain eye contact as you weave your legs around your partner's.

2. Turning toward you, your partner slides the arm closest to you under your waist, holding the base of your spine, lower back, or buttocks. Your partner then places the other hand on your neck or shoulders, firmly kneading and pressing the muscles with the thumb and fingers.

3. Interlace your fingers, gaze into each other's eyes, and breathe deeply together. Take a deep inhalation, hold it for a few seconds, then exhale slowly together, completely emptying all the air in your lungs. Continue to breathe deeply in sync for a couple of minutes, allowing your breaths to grow long and deep as you absorb the love and energy from each other's eyes. This is a good time to enjoy some alluring, long, slow, gentle, deep kisses.

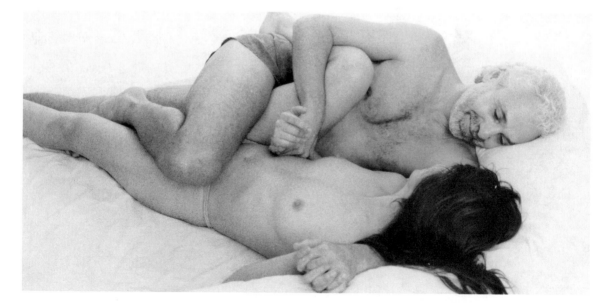

Variation: Gentle Strokes

1. With the hand that was on the abdomen in Step 3 of Romantic Intertwine, lightly stroke your partner's inner thigh, gliding over the Joy of Living point (Lv 9), located on the middle of the inner thigh. Then move up toward Sp 12 and Sp 13, the Rushing Door and Mansion Cottage points in the groin.

2. As you lightly stroke the thigh, your partner can sensitively touch the length of your back, from the base of the spine all the way up to the base of the skull.

Suggestions

- Use your feet to make contact with your partner's feet. Maintain eye contact while having contact with both of your lover's feet will establish a powerful connection. Slowly move your feet until they comfortably fit with your partner's body.

- Play with the amount of space between you, slowly moving a few inches back away from your partner and then gradually coming forward, a little closer together. Notice the different facial features that come into focus, depending upon the distance between your faces, as you continue to gaze into each other's eyes. Feel free to giggle or talk to each other while you maintain direct eye contact.

  The current of energy that circulates from the eyes to the feet balances a couple's minds and bodies. This posture enables you to have satisfying verbal communication while making physical contact, in addition to deep passionate kissing. You may find the intimacy generated from this posture enhances your romantic connection, openness, and affection for making love.

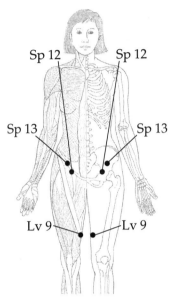

Acupressure Points

Point	Name	Location
CV 24	*Supporting Nourishment*	On the chin, in the depression below the middle of the lower lip
CV 2–CV 6	*Sea of Intimacy*	In the center of the lower abdomen, between the navel and the pubic bone
Sp 12 Sp 13	*Rushing Door* *Mansion Cottage*	Between the hip and pubic bone, in the center of the groin
B 10	*Heavenly Pillar*	One finger-width below the base of the skull, on the ropy muscles one-half inch outward from the spine
TW 15	*Heavenly Rejuvenation*	One-half inch below the top of the shoulder
SI 12–SI 14	*Adaptability Points*	Close to the upper edge of the shoulder blade
GV 20	*One Hundred Meeting*	In the center of the top back of the head
GB 14–GB 21	*Receiving Spirit Points*	On the skull, from the forehead to the base of the skull
GB 30–GB 34	*Jumping Circle Points*	On the outside of the hip and the outer thigh
Lv 8–Lv 12	*Joy of Living*	On the inside of the thigh, from the knee to the groin
K 2–K 7	*Sexual-Reproductive Trigger Points*	On the inside of the ankle and lower leg

Touching the Delights Below

Let your partner rest in your arms. As you caress his or her face, imagine that the pleasure of your touch is melting away any of your partner's stress. Breathe together and hold each other securely, taking refuge in your embrace.

The following couple's exercise is calming, nurturing, and relaxing. When you hold your partner in this position for a few minutes, breathing deeply together, several facial acupressure points will release under your fingertips, bringing greater serenity to your relationship.

Directions

1. With your partner on his or her back, lie down on your side close by. Lean on your elbow, holding your partner's neck muscles for support.

2. Using your upper hand, comfortably position your fingers on your partner's face, applying gentle pressure on points St 3 and LI 21. Hold the points very lightly if your partner finds them tender.

Suggestions

• If your hand gets tired, rest it on your partner's back or shoulders, embracing your love.

• Take long, slow, deep breaths, synchronizing each breath with your partner's. At the top of the inhalation, hold your breath for 5 seconds. Control the flow of air as you exhale, slowing it down. Stay in sync with your partner's breath.

Variations

• **Opening the Sea of Intimacy:** Continue leaning on your elbow, using that hand to firmly support your partner's neck. Squeeze both sides of your partner's neck, using the heel of your hand on one side, your fingertips on the other.

Gradually apply firm pressure with the palm of your other hand into your partner's lower abdomen. Bring the elbow of that arm up high, enabling the weight of your arm and hand to sink into your partner's belly. The Sea of Intimacy points (CV 2–CV 6) in the lower abdominal area are vital for strengthening the reproductive system and increasing energy flow through the pelvis. Breathing deeply into these lower abdominal points enables you to experience greater depths of intimacy and sexual pleasure.

A new commandment I give to you, that you love one another.

—Jesus

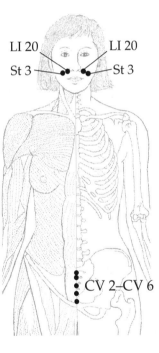

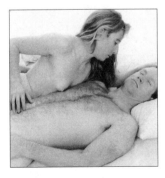

145

- **Tantalizing the Genitals:** The hand that is on your partner's lower abdomen can slide down to the groin points (Sp 12, Sp 13) and then gradually move to the points of the pubic bone. Lightly stroke and tantalize the encompassing area around the genitals, taking time to enjoy all the sensations. Breathe as slowly and deeply as possible. Visualize the area magnified several times as you consciously caress the upper thighs close to the genitals in an arousing superslow motion. Stay in the moment, and breathe with your partner as you follow your desire for engaging in oral sex or intercourse.

Acupressure Point Stimulation

Facial Points:	St 3, B 2, St 6
Chest Points:	St 13–St 16, K 27, CV 17, Lu 1
Abdominal/Pelvic Points:	CV 2–CV 8, Sp 12, Sp 13
Feet and Ankle Points:	K 2–K 6, Sp 3–Sp 6

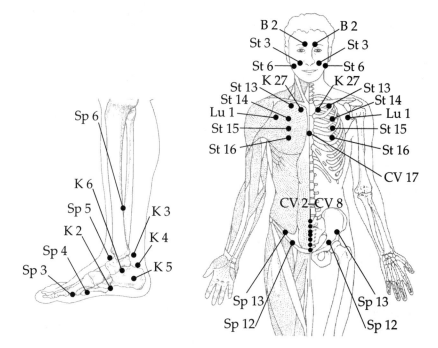

Benefits: This couple's posture has great versatility, from nurturing and calming to stimulating each other's sexual appetites. Holding the points on the face and chest is relaxing, while the points on the abdomen and pelvis have an arousing nature. Experiencing this contrast often brings couples to a new level of intimacy.

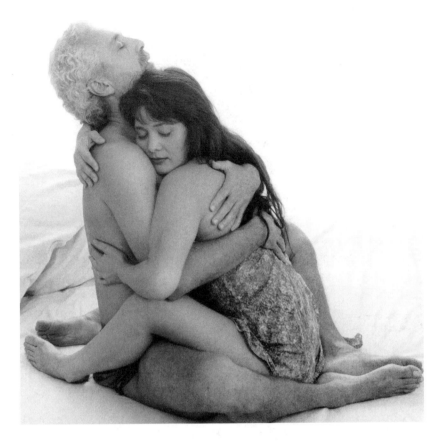

The Seesaw Ride

This is a primary posture used in Tantra rituals for increasing intimacy in lovemaking. The seesaw movement not only creates physical balance between lovers but releases stress and attunes the emotional relationship. Its embraces and movements provide the necessary ingredients for freeing each other's spirits. Being spontaneous and playful is vital for a healthy love relationship.

Caution: This exercise is not for those who have suffered a recent neck injury or have a cervical or lumbar weakness or debilitation.

Directions
1. Consider doing this posture naked, whether or not you choose to be sexual. Wrap your arms and legs around each other, opening your love, bringing your partner into you.

To stay in the sensory present as you make love, remain aware of change. Totally be at the points of contact between skin and skin. Be one, literally, with the sensations themselves. Stay at the intersections of sensory greeting.

—David and Ellen Ramsdale
Sexual Energy Ecstasy

147

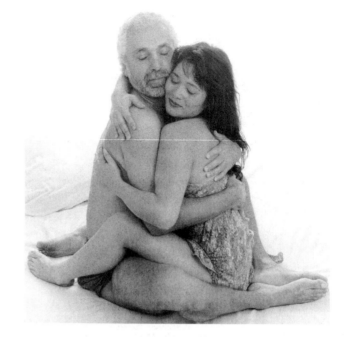

My willingness to be intimate with my own deep feelings creates the space for intimacy with another. Enjoying my own company allows me to have fun with whomever I'm with. And feeling the aliveness and power of the universe flowing through me creates a life of passionate feeling and fulfillment.

—Shakti Gawain
Living in the Light

2. Sit with your legs bent, with the bottoms of your feet together. (If your partner is larger than you are, he or she should sit this way instead.) Your partner sits between your knees, straddling your body. Scoot your pelvis as close as possible to your partner.

3. Comfortably place your arms around each other. Massage and knead each other's back and neck muscles for a couple of minutes.

4. Slowly rock your upper bodies forward and backward. As your partner leans backward, you will naturally be pulled forward.

5. Inhale deeply as you come up and lean back; exhale slowly as you come forward. Enjoy this movement while breathing deeply.

Suggestions

• **Open to the Inner Child:** Explore the Seesaw Ride with your eyes open. Enjoy watching your partner move. Be playful together. When two adults gently play together, feeling safe to free the inner child of long ago, a precious joyous spirit emerges. Play like children—open and new, fully present and carefree.

• **Opening Verbally to Each Other:** The Seesaw is a good position to tell each other verbally what feels right to your bodies. Stay open to your partner's feedback: where to position your hands, how he or she wants to be massaged, and how far back to lean.

Talk or make playful sounds, communicating through the tones of your voice as you rock back and forth. Use the power and sensitivity of your touch to communicate with your partner as well.

• **Massage with Your Eyes Closed:** Make your movements extremely slow so you can fully trust and enjoy your partner's body. Massage each other's back and shoulders. Knead the muscles firmly with your fingertips and thumbs as you slowly rock back and forth, breathing deeply together.

When you want to vary the pattern of your movement or increase the speed, make the change gradually. Your bodies may spontaneously shift into various other movements. For example, try slowly rocking from side to side and then in a circular motion. When the movement begins to shift, slow down again, balancing your bodies' weight. Also fully open your spontaneity.

• **Let Your Body Go:** Seesaw back and forth, in sync with your partner's movements and breathing. As you lean back, take a full deep breath, letting your head relax back. As you exhale and come forward, let yourself completely relax. Continue to move gracefully with your partner while being fully present in the moment. *Note:* People with neck problems should not practice this variation.

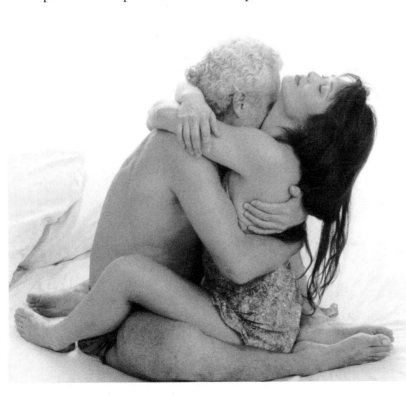

Variations

- **Balancing to See Your Love:** With your arms extended and your fingers curved, hook into your partner's neck, shoulders, or back as you both gently lean backward. Find a balanced position.

  Notice what thoughts surface, what love, sadness, or fear comes up as you gaze into the deep wells of your partner's eyes. After noticing the expressions on your lover's face, talk about what you saw or imagined. If you don't feel like talking, slow your movements down and breathe deeply together as you gaze into each other's eyes.

- **Seesaw Heart Kiss:** Place your hands on your partner's back. As your head comes forward, relax your forehead on his or her breastbone. As you lean back, your partner can place his or her forehead on your breastbone, connecting your Third Eye point (GV 24.5) with the center of your breastbone (CV 17).

  After enjoying this position, you can also kiss CV 17, on the center of the chest. Be sure to slow down your movements, prolong your kiss, and breathe into your heart, feeling the energy flow.

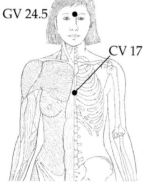

GV 24.5

CV 17

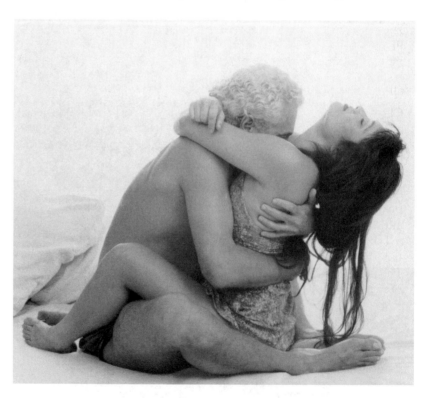

- **Third Eye Kisses:** As your partner lowers his or her head downward, chin toward the chest, bring your lips to the center of the forehead. Breathe deeply through your nose as you kiss your partner's Third Eye point (GV 24.5) on the forehead, using firm suction between the eyebrows. As your hands firmly support the back of your partner's head, awaken the Third Eye with your kiss. A passionate kiss on the lips after stimulating this spiritual point is a wonderfully intimate experience.

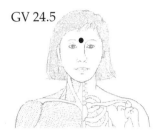

GV 24.5

Advanced Variations

Note: People with lower back or neck problems should not practice the next two advanced variations.

- **Soaring Eagle:** Your partner interlaces his or her fingers behind your lower back, giving you firm support as you slowly lean back for the duration of one deep breath. Tilt your head back, letting your arms stretch out—surrendering and opening like a soaring eagle. Then come forward and relax. After repeating this a couple of times, switch, letting your partner soar.

- **Swaying—Letting Your Tensions Go:** With your hands around your partner's waist, move them up the back, your fingers pointing upward. Curve them to hook onto your partner's shoulders. As you hold the shoulders in this position, let your partner lean all the way backward. Slowly sway your partner from side to side, allowing his or her head to dangle.

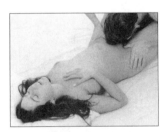

- **Closer to Making Love:** As you continue to rock your bodies back and forth, the partner sitting underneath straightens and spreads his or her legs. Gradually and gracefully lower your partner backward, supporting the lower back until your partner's body reaches the floor or mattress. As you kneel between your partner's legs, slowly lower your body on top of him or her. This new position can lead to a wide range of kissing, massaging, passionate embracing, and eventually oral sex or intercourse.

The Seesaw Ride posture stimulates the three meridians that nourish the sexual-reproductive system: kidney, liver, and spleen. These energy pathways travel through the inner thigh and groin, which are stretched in this exercise. These other points are also strongly stimulated:

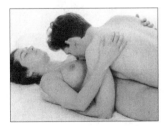

Acupressure Points

Point	Name	Location
B 10	*Heavenly Pillar*	One finger-width below the base of the skull on the ropy muscles, one-half inch outward from the spine
GB 21	*Shoulder Well*	On the top of the shoulder muscle, one to two inches from the side of the lower neck
TW 15	*Heavenly Rejuvenation*	One-half inch below the top of the shoulders, midway between the base of the neck and the outside edge of the shoulder cap
B 38	*Vital Diaphragm*	Between the shoulder blades and the spine, at heart level
B 23, B 47	*Sea of Vitality*	On the lower back, two and four finger-widths away from the spine at waist level, in line with the belly button
CV 17	*Sea of Tranquility*	On the center of the breast-bone, four finger-widths up from the base of the breast-bone
P 6	*Inner Gate*	Three finger-widths above the center of the inner wrist crease, between the tendons
Lv 9	*Joy of Living*	One-third of the way up from the knee toward the inner groin, on the inside of the thigh between the muscles

Benefits: The acupressure points stimulated in the Seesaw Ride relieve lower back stiffness as well as shoulder and neck tension.

Chapter 9

ACUPRESSURE FOR
ORAL SEX

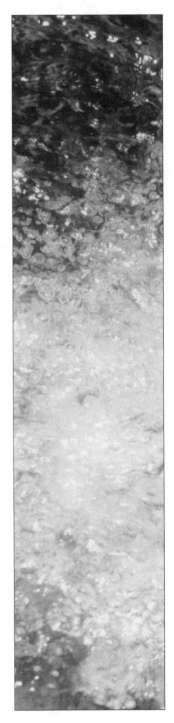

*A*ndy came to me because he was having sexual problems with his wife; he felt nettled by her touch, especially while receiving oral sex. He could give her oral sex, but when she touched him, his body would tense up from sensory overload. I arranged for a series of acupressure sessions, both singly with Andy and jointly with his wife, to show them various points and techniques for relaxing his body.

After two months, Andy told me that the acupressure techniques had helped to alleviate the anxiety he felt about oral sex and being touched during intercourse. He said that his sexual responsiveness was dramatically improved when his wife applied acupressure to his back before and during lovemaking. His progress did not occur overnight, he said, but step by step, as he learned to trust his own body and let go of inner conflicts and performance pressures.

The deep pleasure you can give your partner through oral sex can be extremely erotic and sensual. This ecstatic experience can also become overwhelming. For people like Andy, oral sex can lead to sensory overload and be more painful than pleasurable. This can cause a person to tense against the highly charged sensorial stimulation. Acupressure can neurologically stabilize this hypersensitivity. Without diminishing the erotic sensations, it balances the body's nervous system and enables sexual energy to flow.

POINTS TO USE DURING ORAL SEX

Since oral sex can be intensely tantalizing and sexually delightful, many people are interested in enhancing it without drugs or alcohol. Fortunately, several points in the pelvis, buttocks, and inner thighs cultivate greater sexual awareness and are natural places to hold during oral sex. These points increase the circulation of blood and energy into the pelvis and genitals. As the points release, greater amounts engorge the area.

As you hold the following points during oral sex, your finger pressure creates a grounding cord for your partner to receive greater amounts of pure pleasure. Contact with these points stabilizes the body and gives your lover a sense of security and assurance. The firmness and strength of holding the points balances the tantalizing movements of oral sex.

An oral sex routine using all of the following points would be too lengthy and laborious to practice with spontaneity. Instead, try stimulating a few of these points each time you have oral sex. Return to the points that your partner enjoys most.

Extreme pleasure

brings bashfulness

and languor.

Jade softens,

blossoms droop.

My hairpin hangs

on my sleeve.

My hair flows

down my arms.

—Sung Yu
Third Century B.C.

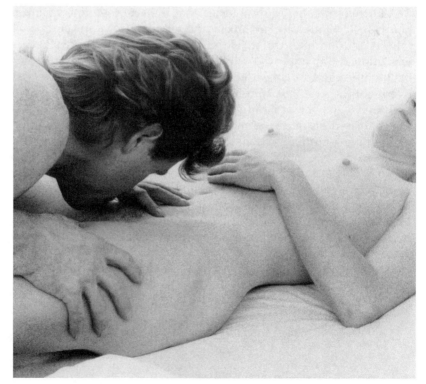

154

Rushing Door (Sp 12) and Mansion Cottage (Sp 13)

Location: In the pelvic area, in the middle of the crease where the leg joins the trunk of the body.

Benefits: Holding these points particularly increases sexual intimacy and enhances sensations in the genitals.

Applications for Oral Sex: In preparation for oral sex, have your partner lie on his or her back. Kneel between your partner's legs. Gently place the heel of your hands on the groin crease where the thigh joins the trunk of the body. With your fingertips lightly on the belly, slowly lean the weight of your chest into your partner's groin points, gradually increasing the pressure. You will feel a strong pulse close to Sp 12 and Sp 13. Adjust your hands for your comfort, and hold for 2 minutes while breathing deeply.

During oral sex, grasp hold of your partner's pelvis, resting the palms of your hands on the base of your lover's hip bone. Rotate your thumbs until they are on the thick ropy band in the groin, halfway between the hip bone and the tip of the pubic bone. Grasping the pelvis firmly with your hands while holding Sp 12 and Sp 13 can be incredibly arousing during oral sex.

For using Rushing Door acupressure points during intercourse, see Chapter 10.

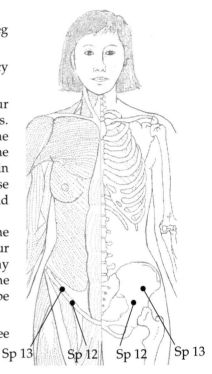

Sp 13   Sp 12   Sp 12   Sp 13

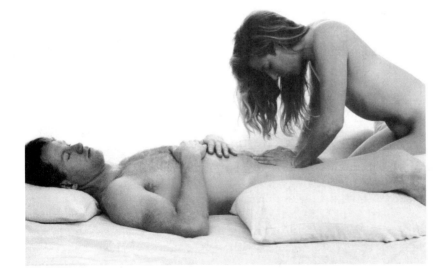

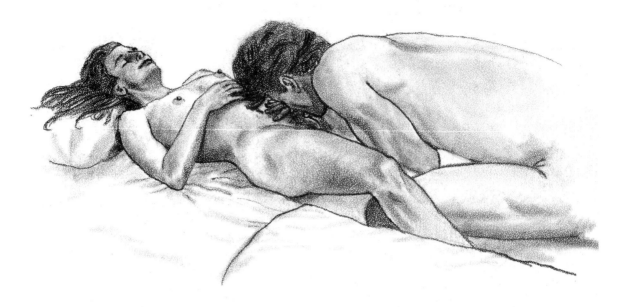

Crooked Bone (CV 2) *and Transverse Bone* (K 11)

Caution: Use these points carefully during pregnancy.

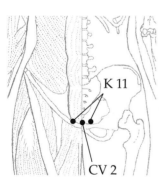

Front View

Location: CV 2 is on the top edge of the pubic bone in the center. (In acupuncture, this point is described as just above the pubic bone. Since a needle would bend if the bone were punctured, the bone is avoided in an acupuncture treatment.) K 11 is half a finger-width from the midline on either side, also on the upper border of the pubic bone.

Benefits: Holding these points increases sexual energy and awareness. It regulates the sexual-reproductive system and helps impotence, spermatorrhea, and pain in the scrotum or penis.

Applications for Cunnilingus: As you kneel between your partner's knees, place your fingertips on CV 2 and K 11 at her pubic bone. Gently use your fingers to draw the skin away from the pubic bone toward the navel to expose the clitoris. First kiss the general area, including the inside of her upper thighs. Then tantalize her vaginal lips, using very slow strokes with your tongue. Gradually encircle the clitoris with the tip of your tongue as you concentrate on breathing slowly and deeply. Once your partner is thoroughly aroused, gently suck on her clitoris.

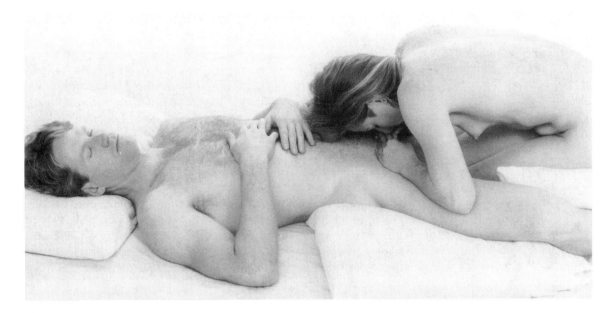

Applications for Fellatio: Kneel between his legs as you gently caress his inner thighs and scrotum. Rest the weight of your hands with the sides of your little fingers on top of your partner's pubic bone, pressing into CV 2 and K 11. Bring the penis upward toward the navel with the pads of your thumbs on top of the exposed shaft. Kiss its entire length. Then lick it like a lollipop until your saliva makes it slippery. Lean some of your weight into these pubic bone points with the sides of your hands and glide the pads of both thumbs up and down the penis as you warm it with your mouth.

When men and women indulge freely in sex, exchanging bodily fluids and breathing each other's breath, it is like fire and water meeting in such perfect proportions that neither one defeats the other.

—Sun-Nu Ching
The Classic of the Plain Girl

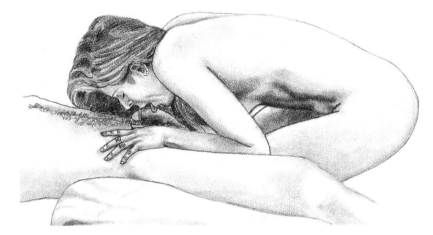

157

Inner Meeting (CV 1)

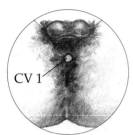

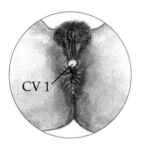

Location: Midway between the anus and genitals.

Benefits: This intimate point enhances orgasm and ejaculation and benefits the reproductive organs. CV 1 has also been used as a revival point, especially for drowning. If I were washed up onto the beach and someone pressed this point on me, I'm sure I would perk up immediately to see what was going on.

Applications for Oral Sex: Your partner is lying on his or her back with knees bent and feet flat on the floor. Kneel or sit on a couple of pillows by your partner's side. Begin by lightly touching the inner thighs and caressing the genitals, encouraging your partner to breathe deeply and spread his or her legs. Place your hand (the hand closest to your partner's feet) under your partner's thigh to press CV 1. Feel for a ropy cordlike structure under the surface of the skin. Place the palm of your other hand on your partner's pubic bone. Lower your head and enjoy giving your lover pleasure.

For other uses of this acupressure point, see the Vitality Saver in Chapter 10 and Erotic Oral Sex later in this chapter.

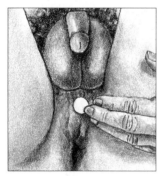

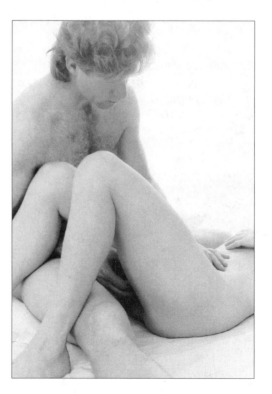

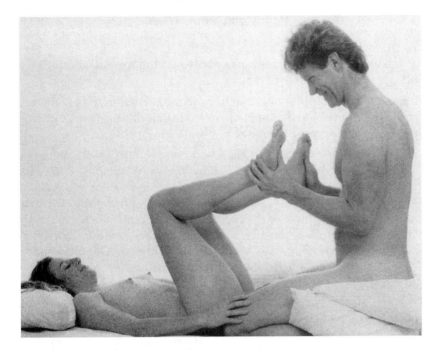

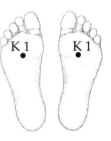

Bubbling Spring (K 1)

Location: On the center of the sole of the foot, at the base of the ball of the foot, between the two pads.

Benefits: This is a powerful point to hold with your thumbs during oral sex when your partner is on his or her back, legs apart with knees bent. Holding it also relieves male and female reproductive system problems such as hot flashes, infertility, scrotal pain, and impotence.

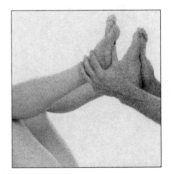

Applications for Oral Sex: With your partner lying on his or her back with knees bent and feet on the floor, kneel between his or her legs. You may find it more comfortable to place a pillow between your heels and buttocks. Bring your partner's knees up toward his or her chest and slide your hands down to the feet. Place the palms of your hands on the outsides of the feet, using your thumbs to press K 1 on the center of the sole of the foot. Use gentle-to-firm pressure, depending upon your partner's sensitivity at this point. Slowly bring your head down toward the genitals to give your lover a creative erotic experience.

Use the Mutual Foot Massage in Chapter 8 to stimulate this point while you give each other a foot massage.

Womb and Vitals (B 48)

Location: 1 to 2 finger-widths outside the sacrum (the large bony area at the base of the spine), midway between the top of the hip bone (iliac crest) and the base of the buttocks.

Benefits: Holding the Womb and Vitals points strongly benefits the sexual-reproductive system. It increases circulation through the pelvis, nurturing your lover's womb and reproductive organs.

Applications for Oral Sex: When you grasp hold of your partner's "love handles" during oral sex, you instinctively stimulate B 48 with your fingertips. As you gradually move closer to your lover's body to give oral sex, press on the outside of his or her buttocks, into the base of the spine at the level of the hips. Since the Womb and Vitals points are located underneath the large muscles of the buttocks, they often need deeper pressure than your fingers can give. Thus, try using either the heel of your hands or the knuckles of your fist, gradually applying pressure into these points during oral sex.

The couple's exercise Riding Your Lover in Chapter 8 stimulates the Womb and Vitals points.

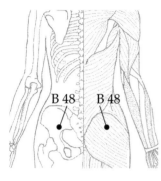

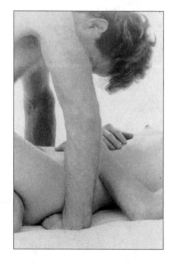

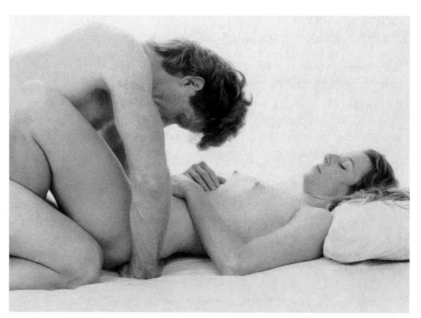

Inner Thigh (Lv 10–Lv 12)

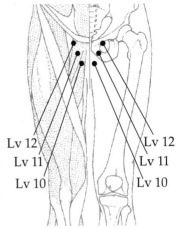

Lv 12   Lv 12
Lv 11   Lv 11
Lv 10   Lv 10

Location: On the inside of the upper thigh, close to the inner crease where the thigh joins the trunk of the body.

Benefits: These points are incredibly sensitive and arousing for lovers to hold and caress. They increase the circulation into the reproductive organs, heightening sensitivity and awareness in the genital region.

Applications for Oral Sex: Lightly stroke Lv 10, Lv 11, and Lv 12 in that order while gazing into your partner's eyes. Lovers find these points to be especially responsive to gentle licks and kisses. Tantalize the area this way as a powerful prelude to oral sex.

You can also hold or fondle these points during oral sex to increase your partner's pleasure.

For using these points to arouse a man, see Chapter 7.

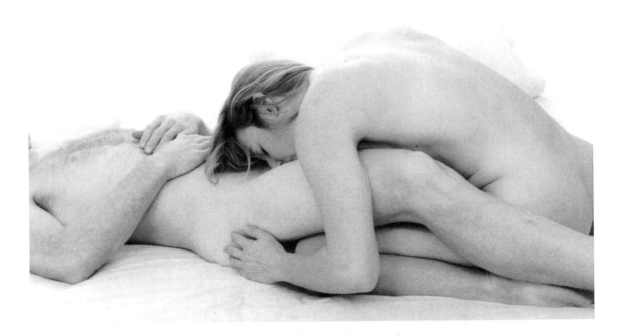

Sacral Points (B 27–B 34)

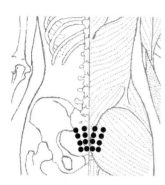

B 27–B 34

Location: On the base of the spine, in the hollows of the sacrum.

Benefits: Steady, firm pressure on these sacral points increases genital pleasure for both men and women during oral sex.

Applications for Oral Sex: With the fingertips of both hands, firmly hold in the slight indentations of the sacral bone for at least 2 minutes during oral sex. As you gradually apply firm pressure to these points, bring your partner's pelvis closer to you, giving stronger stimulation and greater pleasure.

Many other applications throughout this book use these points. A couple's exercise that strongly stimulates them is called Riding Your Lover in Chapter 8.

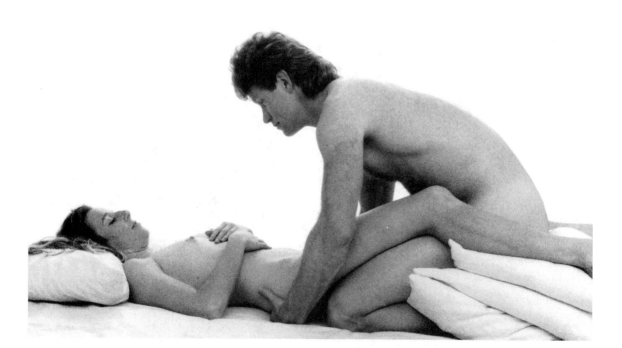

Sea of Vitality (B 23 and B 47)

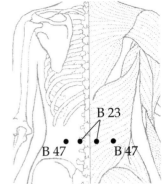

Caution: Do not press on disintegrating disks or fractured bones. If you have a weak back, use light touching instead of pressure. See your doctor first if you have questions or need medical advice.

Location: On the lower back 2 and 4 finger-widths away from the spine at waist level, in line with the belly button.

Benefits: Hold these points for relieving sexual-reproductive problems, impotence, and premature ejaculation.

Applications for Oral Sex: During oral sex, place one of your hands on the lower back, positioning your other hand over that hand for support. Firmly squeeze the ropelike muscular cords on both sides, using your fingertips and the heel of your hand for 1 or 2 minutes.

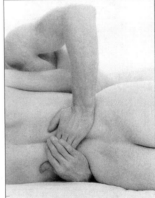

These points are powerfully stimulated in: Soaring Eagle, the advanced variation on the Seesaw Ride from Chapter 8, and the Mutual Massage in the Lovemaking Progressions in Chapter 10.

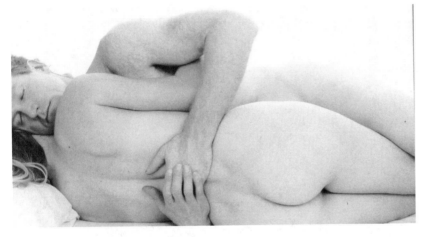

ORAL SEX POINT SUMMARY

Experiment with different ways of holding these oral sex points. Try using your thumbs as well as your fingertips for each point. As you adjust your body and your hands, creating different ways of approaching these points, continue to ask your partner what feels best. Enjoy exploring and learning about yourselves!

LOVE PROGRESSIONS LEADING TO ORAL SEX

When life is hurried and frenetic, we often have difficulty finding the time to share thoughtful lovemaking with our partner. In order to maintain the quality of a relationship, actions must be balanced with repose. The following posture is especially nurturing in a love relationship, as it deeply relaxes you and attunes you to your partner.

Directions

1. Take some time at the end of your day to relax and reflect with your partner. Lie down on your sides, facing each other and cuddling close. Close your eyes and take several deep breaths together before you talk.

2. As your partner slowly rolls onto his or her back, with legs slightly spread, lean forward and gently rest the side of your head on the center of your lover's chest as a pillow.

3. Place one hand on your partner's neck or head, and place the palm of the other hand on the center of the lower abdomen, midway between the navel and the pubic bone (CV 2–CV 6).

4. Bring your upper leg over your partner's thigh, placing the arch of your foot comfortably on top of your partner's foot.

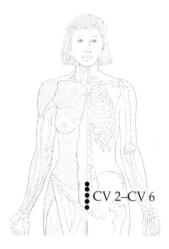

CV 2–CV 6

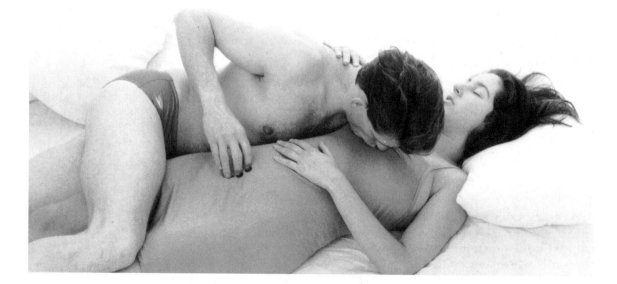

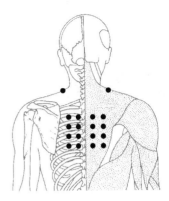

5. Meanwhile, your partner firmly holds acupressure points on your upper back. Find the large ropy muscles between your shoulder blades with the hand in back of you. Meanwhile his or her hand in front massages your shoulders or temples.

Suggestions

- Hook into the points. Have your partner curve his or her fingers, firmly hooking into the muscles of the upper back, shoulders, and neck.

- Breathe simultaneously, slowly and deeply into your hearts, as you embrace each other. Breathe in the love you feel for each other. Hold your breath for about 5 seconds at the top of the inhalation to feel the fullness of your energy. Let yourself go, and completely relax as you exhale, merging deeper and deeper into your lover. Breathe deeply, and allow the tensions of the day to dissipate.

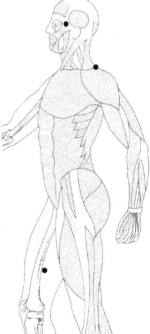

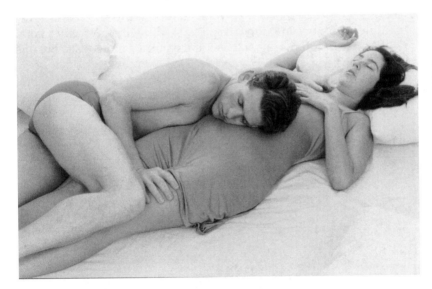

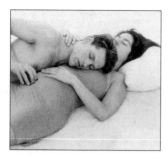

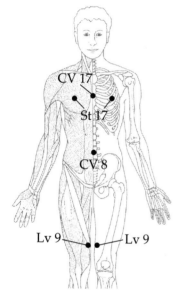

Variations

- **Kiss point CV 17,** on the middle of the breastbone. Then place your ear on the center of the breastbone on CV 17, level with your partner's heart. Continue with the deep breathing as you listen to your partner's heart.

- **Suck your partner's nipples,** stimulating point St 17. As you move your head down, resting it on the navel (CV 8), your hand moves from your partner's neck or head to the temples, shoulders, or lower back. Your other hand can slowly and lightly caress the inner thigh, starting at the middle of the inner thigh (Lv 9, the Joy of Living point). Sensually glide toward the genitals several times. The points in the groin stimulate sexual energy. Encourage your partner to breathe deeply with you.

- **Touch the Sea of Love.** The hand that was at your partner's temples or shoulder moves down to the nipple (St 17). Roll it between your fingertips as you gaze into your partner's eyes. Maintaining contact with the nipples, use your other hand to reach under the back of your partner's upper thigh to hold the Inner Meeting point (CV 1), pressing midway between the rectum and genitals. Breathe deeply together in sync.

  Bring your face down close to the pubic bone, Sea of Love, surrounding your lover's genitals. After holding the Inner Meeting point, let yourself be erotic, slowly caressing with a silky, gentle touch arousal points not mapped out on any acupressure charts. Lightly use your hands, lips, and tongue to tantalize the whole genital area with the utmost slowness.

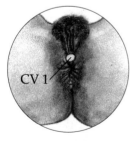

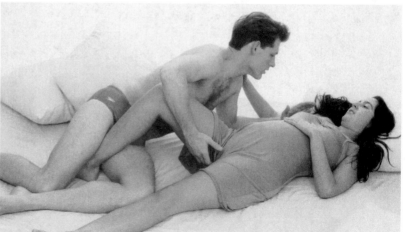

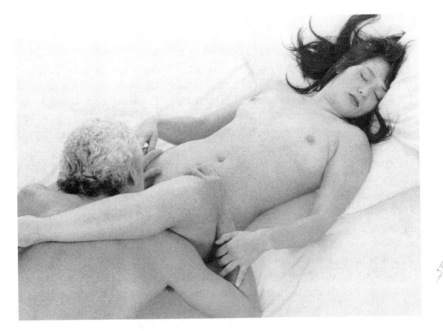

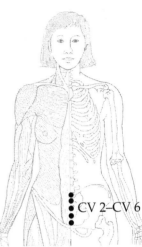

CV 2–CV 6

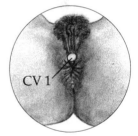

CV 1

Oral Sex on a Woman

As you continue to gently touch the genital area, your partner's legs will naturally open as she relaxes. Raise the leg that is closest to you, positioning yourself between her legs, draping her uplifted leg on your back. Gently rest your forehead on her pelvic bone to press CV 2 while you explore with slow movements with your nose. Try holding these points while you give your partner pleasure with your tongue:

- Place the fingertips of one hand just above the center of her pubic bone on CV 2–CV 6. Gently use your fingers to draw the skin away from the pubic bone toward her navel. Your other hand can lightly stroke the anal area or the inner thighs, or caress the CV 1 point between the vagina and anus.

- Place both of your hands under her buttocks, and use your fingers to press the acupressure points on the base of the spine (B 27–B 34).

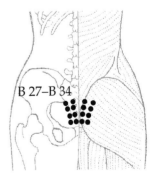

B 27–B 34

Oral Sex on a Man

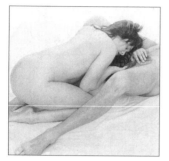

As you reposition your body, kneeling between your partner's legs, gently caress his inner thighs and scrotum. Press Lv 10–Lv 12 on the upper inner thigh with your thumbs. Bring the penis upward toward the navel, kissing the exposed underside. Begin licking it, using your saliva to make it slippery. Press CV 1, midway between the anus and scrotum, as you slide your tongue or the fingers of your other hand up and down the full length of the shaft.

Reposition your body, turning around to face his toes and straddle his waist. Gently sit on his lower belly. Your buttocks will be pressing a series of acupressure points that open sexual energy (CV 2–CV 6, K 12–K 16, and St 26–St 29). Caress the length of the penis again, wrapping the fingers of both of your hands around it and securely forming a double ring. As you bring your mouth around the head, coat it with more saliva or a natural lubricant. (Kama Sutra's Oil of Love is an excellent natural lubricant that warms the skin erotically.) Move up and down the penis with your mouth, building speed.

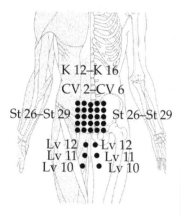

CV 1

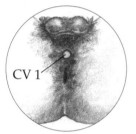

K 12–K 16
CV 2–CV 6
St 26–St 29   St 26–St 29
Lv 12 • • Lv 12
Lv 11 • • Lv 11
Lv 10 • • Lv 10

Front View

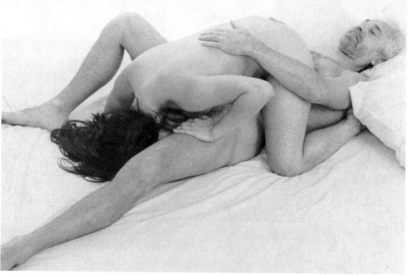

Acupressure Points

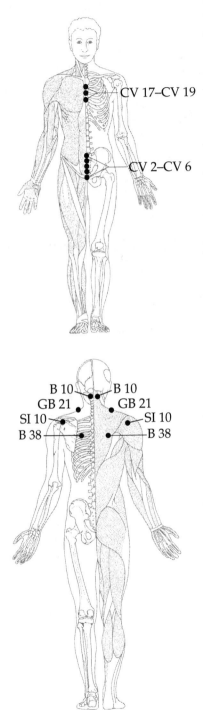

Point	Name	Location
B 10	*Heavenly Pillar*	One finger-width below the base of the skull, on the ropy muscles, one-half inch outward from the spine
GB 21	*Shoulder Well*	On the highest point of the top of the shoulder muscle, 1 to 2 finger-widths down from the side of the neck
SI 10	*Shoulder Blade*	In the joint of the shoulder, where the upper arm bone meets the shoulder blade
B 38	*Vital Diaphragm*	Between the shoulder blade and the spine, at heart level
CV 17– CV 19	*Sea of Tranquility*	On the center midline, in the indentations of the breastbone
CV 2– CV 6	*Sea of Intimacy*	In the center of the lower abdomen, between the navel and the the pubic bone
CV 1	*Inner Meeting*	Midway between the anus and the genitals

Benefits: The postures in this chapter nourish the heart, calm the spirit, and recharge a couple's batteries through deep relaxation and sexual arousal.

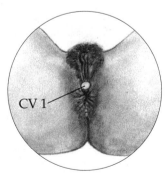

CV 1

EMBRACING LOVE

The following positions, movements, and acupressure points can heighten sexual arousal. The experience they give you will vary greatly depending upon your intention and mood, whether your clothes are on or off, and whether your eyes are open or closed. Begin by talking to your lover. Determine whether you are in the mood for being sexual, who wants to give, and who wants to receive.

Directions

1. Your lover lies down on his or her back, knees bent, feet flat on the floor, arms comfortably resting at his or her side.

2. Kneel in front of your partner's feet.

3. With your hands on the recipient's knees, slowly lean forward, bringing your partner's knees into his or her chest. The knees can be together or apart. Slowly rock the knees in toward the chest as your partner exhales. This stretches your partner's legs, opens the pelvis, and gently stretches the lower back. As you release the pressure and rock back, your partner inhales, visualizing a wave washing up on the sand and returning to a calm bay.

It's not just giving that brings pleasure; it's also receiving. In concert, these two essential human acts join in a circle of interaction that expands with use. When the circle is complete, the more you give, the more you get, and vice versa.

—George Leonard

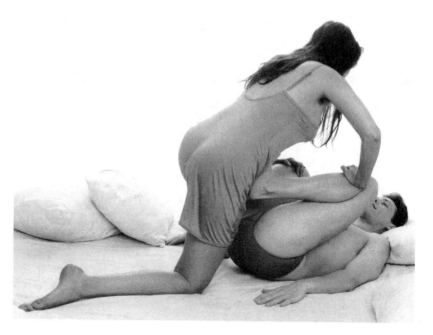

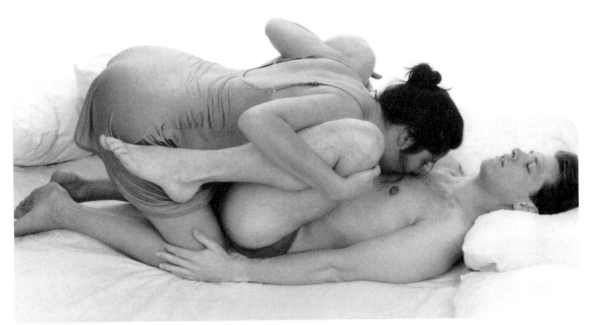

4. Spread your partner's knees apart slowly. With your upper body between his or her knees, grasp the outside of the legs. As you hug your partner's legs, slowly rock your upper body back and forth. During this movement you can hold on to your partner's knees or thighs. Stimulate the series of points in the center of the body, from the heart down to the pubic bone, by gradually rolling your head over your partner's chest and belly. If your partner's clothes are off, you can also stimulate the points by kissing.

5. Gradually lean forward to kiss the heart center, the Sea of Tranquility point (CV 17), on the breastbone directly between the nipples. Apply some suction or a comfortable amount of body weight as you continue to kiss the center of the breastbone.

6. Slowly progress down the center of the body with your kisses, from the breastbone through the navel to the pubic bone. This playful teasing, gentle touching, and licking can lead to passionate sexual arousal.

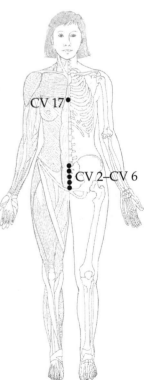

171

There is one way of breathing that is shameful and constricted. Then there's another way: a breath of love that takes you all the way to infinity.

—Rumi
Open Secret

Suggestions

• Make all of your movements slow and graceful.

• Pay close attention to how your partner is breathing for feedback. If the breathing is slow and deep, then your partner is relaxing. Shallow breathing may mean that your partner is not fully participating in the experience. To engage your partner more, encourage him or her to breathe deeply with you.

• Place your hands underneath your partner's buttocks, firmly pulling the pelvis in toward your chest. Drape the legs over your shoulders. Focus on breathing deeply together while you gently play with slow movements, kisses, and gentle touch.

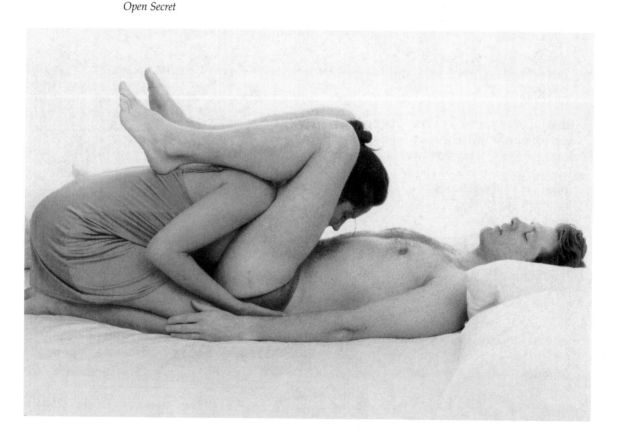

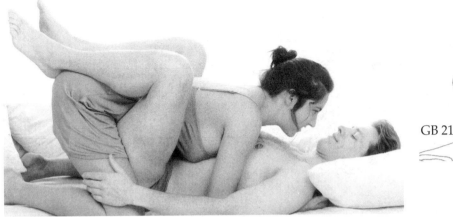

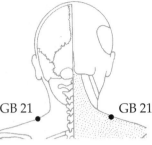

GB 21   GB 21

Massage Variations

- **Embracing the Shoulders:** Gently slide your hands up to the top of your partner's shoulders (GB 21). Curve your fingers, and gradually apply firm finger pressure on the tightest muscles of the shoulders. Embrace your partner with the love you share together.

- **Sit Bone Palace:** In the same position, scoot your knees away from your partner. Use the flat padding of your thumbs to gradually press the soft tissue around your partner's sit bones, anus, and inner thigh. Lean your body weight into your thumbs, and avoid pressing on bone. This variation is especially good for the prostate gland and it can also be very pleasurable.

When you really relax while making love and don't make the usual orgasm your goal, you become available to a grand new brand of sexual peak experiences.

—David and Ellen Ramsdale
Sexual Energy Ecstasy

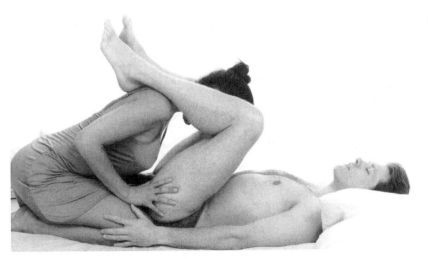

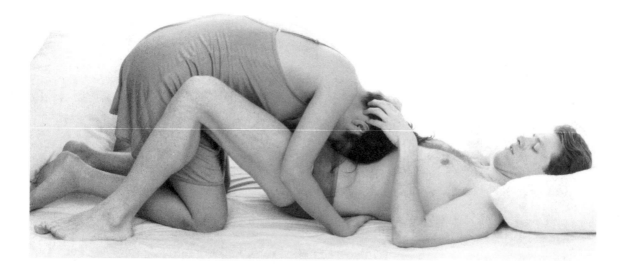

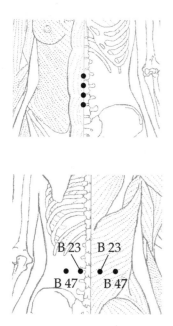

- **Abdominal Head Massage:** Your partner places his or her feet flat on the floor on either side of you. As your partner lifts his or her pelvis up, place one hand all the way underneath the lower back, at the level of the waist, with your fingers pressing on one side of the lower back muscles and the heel of your hand pressing on the other. Place your other hand under that hand for firm support. As your partner lowers his or her back onto your curved fingers, lean toward him or her, applying firm pressure on both sides of the lower back.

Remain in this hand position and gently place the top of your head on your partner's belly. Using utmost care, slowly rock your head over the abdomen. Ask for feedback. If it hurts, simply reduce the amount of pressure and move more slowly. It's a good sign if your partner says that it "hurts good." Be careful not to overdue this abdominal massage—1 minute is more than enough time.

Caution: This abdominal head rocking massage should not be practiced on a pregnant or menstruating woman or on a person with a chronic or serious illness, such as heart disease, cancer, or high blood pressure, or of course if your partner has just eaten beans.

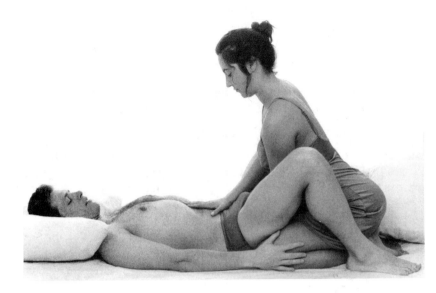

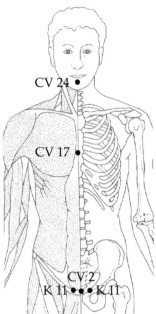

• **Sexually Arousing Your Lover:** Again, as your partner lifts his or her pelvis up, place one hand underneath your partner's sacrum, at the base of the spine. Your other hand holds the lower abdomen, with the heel of your hand on the pubic bone (K 11, CV 2). These sacral points can trigger a strong connection with the genitals, stimulating your partner's sexual energy. Feel free to gently bite, lick, and suck your lover's inner thighs.

Another sexually arousing technique is to place the flat portion of your upper chin so that your CV 24 (just below your lower lip) presses the top of your partner's pubic bone (K 11 and CV 2). Place your hands underneath your partner's buttocks, between the legs.

A couple who can make love ecstatically together are likely to provide each other with peace and harmony in every way and hence their loving attraction for each other may increase and become a more permanent one.

—Jolan Chang
The Tao of Love and Sex

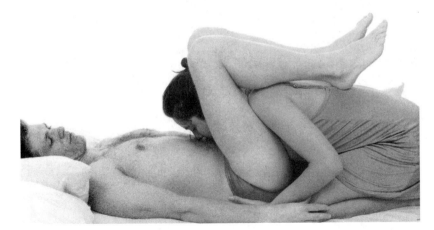

175

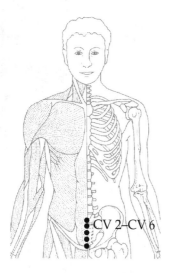

CV 2–CV 6

Orgasm may be the movement of ecstasy when two people soar along a Milky Way among stars all their own. This moment is the high mountaintop of love over which the poets sing, on which the two together become a full orchestra playing a fortissimo of a glorious symphony.

—Lionel Lewis and
Daniel Brissett
Sex as Work

Slowly but firmly knead your partner's buttocks. Keep your eyes closed and breathe deeply. After a few minutes of kneading, when the buttocks are thoroughly relaxed, turn your head to the side, resting it on your partner's belly.

Comfortably reposition your bodies, bringing your arms around the outside of the hips. Place your hands under the sacrum at the base of the spine. Then place the center of your breastbone (CV 17) on top of your partner's pubic bone (CV 2, K 11). Using this contact of breast and pubic bones as a fulcrum, rock your lover's pelvis, either in circles or side to side, breathing slowly and deeply all the while. Your partner can massage your head, resting on its side, while you embrace your partner's pelvic area. Rest in this position, synchronizing your breathing.

Kiss and suck the Conception Vessel points starting at CV 6, the Sea of Intimacy. Work your way down to CV 5, CV 4, and CV 3, then eventually to CV 2 and the area surrounding your partner's genitals. Bring both of your hands ever so gently to this area. Once your partner seems fully aroused, thoroughly enjoy licking the heart of your partner's pleasure.

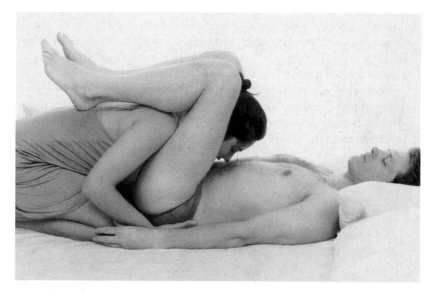

Acupressure Points

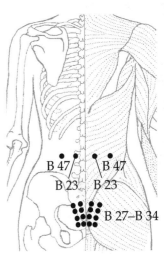

Point	Name	Location
B 23, B 47	*Sea of Vitality*	In the lower back, 2 and 4 finger-widths away from the spine, at the level of the waist
B 27, B 28	*Small Intestine and Bladder Correspondence*	On the base of the spine, directly above the tailbone
B 29, B 30	*Mid-back and Anal Sphincter Correspondence*	On the sacrum, at the base of the spine
B 31, B 32	*Upper Sacral Bones*	On the sacrum, at the base of the spine
B 33, B 34	*Mid- and Lower Sacral Bones*	On the sacrum, at the base of the spine
CV 17	*Sea of Tranquility*	On the center of the breastbone, in the indentation 4 finger-widths up from the base of the breastbone
CV 2–CV 6	*Sea of Intimacy*	In the lower abdomen, between the navel and pubic bones

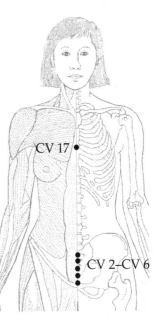

Benefits: In addition to being sexually arousing, the movements in this position gently stretch the lower back, groin, and legs. Regular practice of this position can also strengthen the eliminative and sexual reproductive organs. The stretches and acupressure points can relieve cold feet, low sexual desire, impotence, infertility, and they can open a frozen, rigid pelvis. As you continue to practice Embracing Love and open your pelvic areas, more erotic feelings, intimacy, and pleasures can merge.

177

EROTIC ORAL SEX

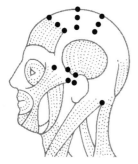

Wash each other's feet in warm water before you begin this lovemaking progression. Move slowly from one position to another.

Sit with your left thighs together, your legs bent outward. Bring your knee close to your partner's hip and vice versa. Bringing your temples together, hug your partner, using your arm muscles to embrace fully. As you hug, move your upper body in slow motion to readjust your bodies until they feel comfortable and your chests fit together. Then mutually massage your partner's back and shoulders.

Take long, deep breaths with your eyes closed as you breathe slowly into each other's ears, giving firm pressure to the temple area.

Loving, rather than being occasional and explosive, is continuous and flowing. Love making should be like a good dinner. Each course should be exquisite in itself and, at the same time, should whet the appetite for the next dish until, at the end of the meal, you are fully satisfied.

—Jolan Chang
The Tao of Love and Sex

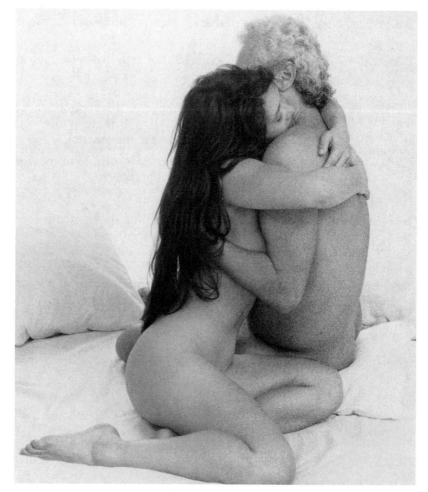

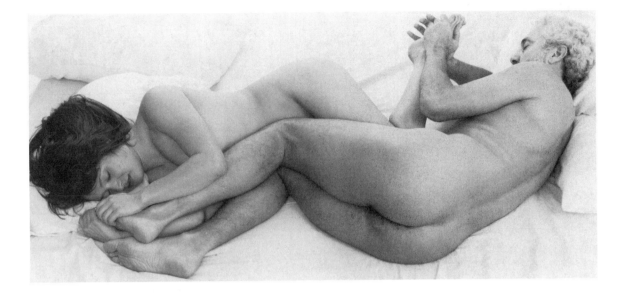

Body Curl

This inverted spooning position enables you to cuddle, stroke each other's legs, and give a wonderful foot massage.

Begin with your clothes off. Lie down on your left sides, head to toe, facing each other with the tops of your thighs touching. (If one partner has a bad left side, then both partners lie on their right side.) Curl up close together, resting on your left elbow. Place a pillow underneath your head to make yourself more comfortable.

Using both of your hands, with your fingers between the bones on the top of the foot and your thumbs on the pads, knead the whole whole length of the top of the foot. Firm pressure will naturally stimulate many foot reflexology and acupressure points.

Once you've completed the top foot, gently push it forward to work on your partner's other foot. Be sure to firmly knead the Achilles tendon and the heels, where many acupressure points are located corresponding to the sexual-reproductive system.

Variation: Hands-On Simon Says

Choose one partner to be the giver, the other the receiver. The giver massages the receiver's foot in the way the giver wants his or her foot massaged, like a nonverbal Simon Says game. The receiver immediately copies the way his or her partner is giving the foot massage. Thus, the giver can communicate hands-on preferences while giving and receiving at the same time. After a few minutes, switch roles.

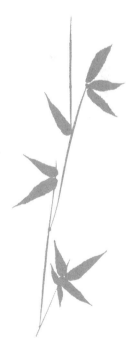

179

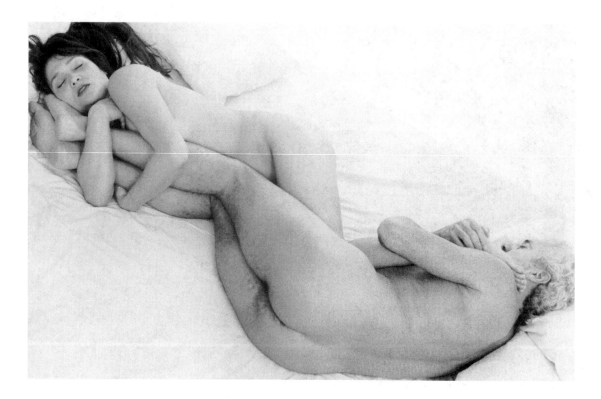

Leg Hug

In the Body Curl position, embrace your partner's lower legs against your chest. Breathe slowly and deeply, hugging your partner's legs firmly.

Toe Suck

Gently bite or suck each toe. Since most of the acupressure pathways either begin or end at the toes or fingertips, you will be stimulating many important points. If you find that using your mouth is awkward or uncomfortable, simply use your fingers to massage the length of each toe, working your fingertips up to the base of the nails where the acupressure points are located.

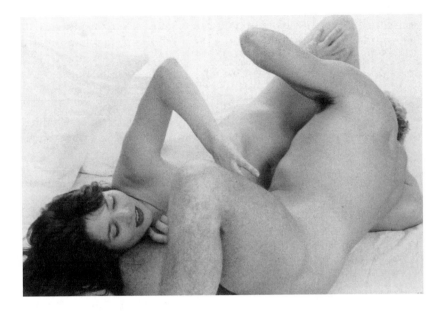

Sixty-nine

Bend your upper leg, placing the bottom of that foot on the floor. This position exposes your genitals. Slowly slide your bodies down, resting the side of your head on the inside of your partner's lower thigh. Your lower leg should be resting on the floor, bent at the knee.

Reposition your bodies until they fit together comfortably. With the fingertips of your right hand, lightly stroke the inside of your partner's right thigh; or use your left hand to stroke your partner's left thigh and calves. Gently tantalize the length of the inner thigh, coming closer and closer to your partner's genitals. Softly caress so that your touch feels like silk. Enjoy the moment, and anticipate the incredible feelings to come.

Slowly bring your head closer and closer to your partner's genitals as you lightly stroke around the anus and genitals, softly gliding over the hairs that grow here. As you continue to fondle the region, kiss around your partner's genitals.

If your partner is a man, caress his scrotum with your fingertips while licking his penis with the flat portion of your tongue. CV 1 is a very satisfying point to hold for channeling male sexual energy. With your other hand, create a magic O by touching your fingertips to the tip of your thumb. Stroke the full length of the penis using the magic O while tantalizing the scrotum and base of the penis with your tongue, lips, and mouth.

She takes off her gauze skirt and loosens his embroidered trousers. Her eyebrows are like a bouquet of flowers; her waist is like a roll of silk. With tender passion she stretches out furtively, and she gazes coyly at her own body. They first pat and knead their flexed bodies, and caress each other from head to toe.

—Po Hsing-chien
Ninth-century Erotic Essay

181

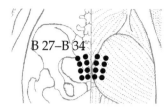

B 27–B 34

The height of sexual love is one of the most total experiences of relationship of which we are capable . . . What lovers feel for each other in this moment is no other than adoration in its full religious sense, and its climax is almost literally the pouring of their lives into each other.

—Alan Watts
Sex as a Contemplative Activity

If your partner is a woman, you can awaken layers of pleasure in her vaginal lips with your tongue. While holding the acupressure points on her sacrum (B 27–B 34), slowly circulate your tongue around her clitoris. There is no rush—take your time. Continue to make slow circles, large and small, until her passion reaches an ecstatic high. Then slowly and gently suck her clitoris.

Savor each moment. Breathe deeply into each sensation. Channel the pleasures you receive by passionately licking, kissing, and sucking. Open yourselves to waves of energy and pleasure.

Benefits: The foot massage, toe suck, and full-body hug of the Body Curl stimulate healing energies. When you relax in the Body Curl or Leg Hug, you may experience a release of energy, much like the afterglow of making love. This double reflexology foot massage stimulates the nerve endings that benefit the internal organs. It is also a great posture to relax and talk with your partner—except when your partner's toe is in your mouth!

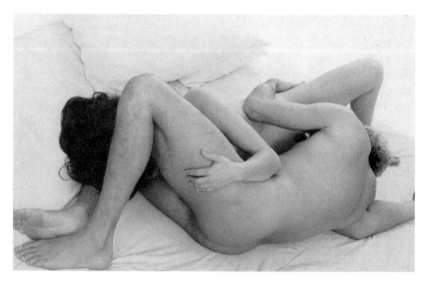

A RECONNECTING COUPLE'S ROUTINE

This routine is a nice way to reconnect with your partner after a long day's work. After a wonderful foot massage, the routine stretches your partner's lower back in an intimate position. Finally you will lie down together in a full-body embrace, a sequence that naturally leads to oral sex or other ways of making love.

1. Foot Massage

Sit facing each other with your legs a shoulder-width apart. Place one leg between your partner's legs. Each partner should grasp hold of the foot that is closest to them and begin massaging the area between the heel and the ankle bones on both sides of the foot. This massage stimulates the acupressure and reflexology points for the reproductive system. Then massage toward the toes, with the thumbs on the top of the foot, fingers on the bottom. Knead the foot as you watch your partner's response. While massaging the feet, you may want to talk or listen to music as you enjoy each other's company.

Bring one hand underneath the ankle and grasp the Achilles tendon, while the other hand kneads the outside of the foot. Then roll each toe while using your other hand to massage the Achilles tendon, the heel, the arch, and the ball of the foot.

Slide your thumb and index finger up and down the large toe as you breathe deeply together, stimulating important energy points for enhancing your sexuality. After finishing one foot, switch your position to massage the other foot, bringing it between your legs. Continue to massage this foot as previously described, until both feet feel equally worked on and balanced.

Be open to experiencing a different form of sexuality than usual; the energy may lead you into simply sitting together, lying together, holding each other, massaging one another, or something else that you don't ordinarily think of as sex but which can be just as satisfying.

—Shakti Gawain
Living in the Light

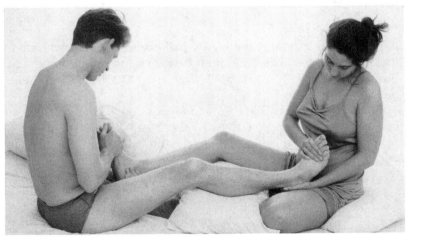

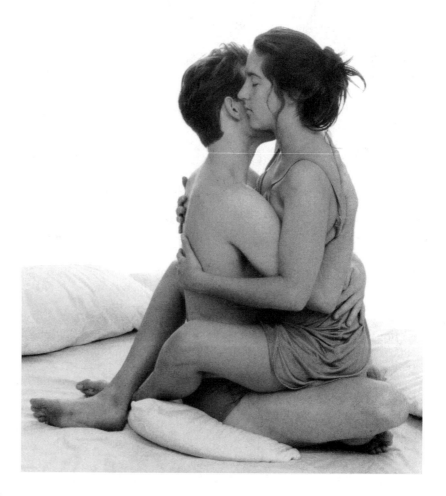

When touching

or being touched,

make that touch

fill all awareness

in that moment.

That touch, or, more

precisely, the field

of sensitivity where

toucher and touched

intercept to create

touching, is the

total universe.

—David and Ellen
Ramsdale
Sexual Energy Ecstasy

2. A Sitting Embrace

After the foot massage, the bigger or heavier partner comfortably crosses his or her legs. The lighter partner sits in the other's lap. Firmly and securely wrap both your arms and legs around each other's backs.

Slowly rock your bodies back and forth as you embrace each other, breathing long and deep into each other's ears. Make sure that your breath is slow and deep as you stretch your bodies and massage each other's backs for a couple of minutes.

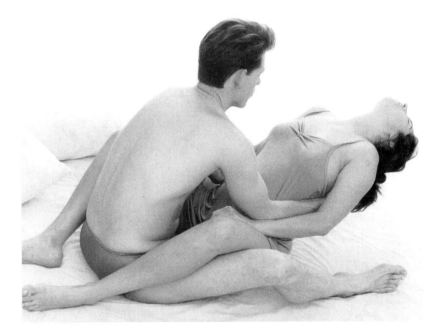

3. Coming Down

As you lean back, your partner firmly holds your shoulders and slowly lowers you down onto your back. Your partner then kneels between your legs and caresses your inner thighs. When you begin breathing rapidly, showing your desire to be touched sexually, your partner can use any of the points mentioned earlier in this chapter while giving you oral sex.

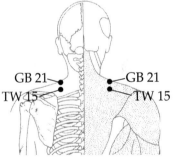

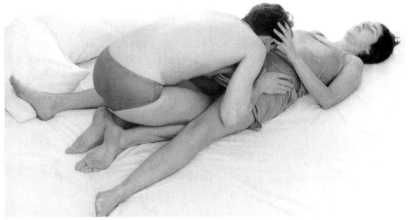

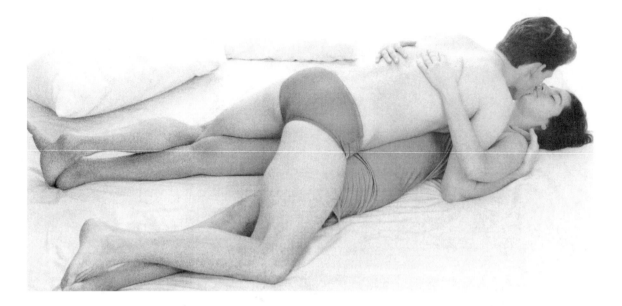

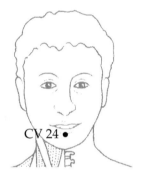

CV 24 •

After licking and sucking, your partner can reposition his or her body by gently lying on top of you. Bend your legs, resting your outer ankle bone in the crease behind your partner's knees or place the tops of your feet against your partner's arches. Place your hands over your partner's lower back, supporting the muscles firmly. Close your eyes as your partner gently presses his or her chin onto the acupressure point (CV 24) between your lower lip and chin. Your partner can also use his or her lips to strongly suck this erotic point.

Continue to breathe deeply as your partner slowly but firmly massages your entire skull and kisses lightly around this chin point. Feel free to rhythmically thrust your pelvis and chest into your partner and surrender your body to the flow of energy.

Breathe deeply into your lover's body. Take in the smells, sounds, and feelings as you express yourself through the magical world of touch. Instead of being driven by your expectations of what should happen, let go, and appreciate the flow you have with each other. Enjoy making love with your whole body.

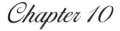

Chapter 10

ACUPRESSURE FOR INTERCOURSE

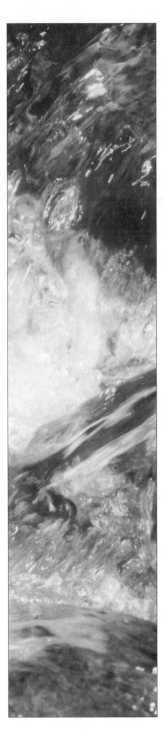

*T*his chapter will show you points and positions that enhance intercourse. First you will learn the major points that your bodies press while making love. Second, you will learn the most potent points to grasp, hold, and press with your hands while you make love. Then you will explore a variety of Lovemaking Progressions, or series of erotic practices that lead to intercourse.

POINTS YOUR BODY PRESSES DURING INTERCOURSE

Some of the points suggested here for intercourse were also recommended for oral sex, as they are gateways for opening the flow of sexual energy and increase blood circulation throughout the pelvic region, particularly into the genitals. When your sexual organs are engorged with nutritious blood, they pulsate and tingle with aliveness, radiating a healthy glow.

When your bodies move and fit together, they stimulate each other's healing energy by stimulating acupressure points. The points on your pubic bone, on your groin, and on the inside of your thighs are naturally stimulated by the posture and movements of lovemaking. Front-to-front intercourse postures activate these primary points.

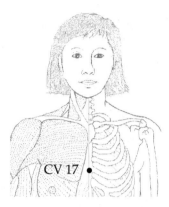

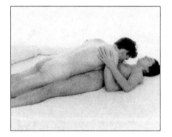

Sea of Tranquility (CV 17)

Location: On the center of the breastbone, four finger-widths up from the base of the bone.

Benefits: Holding this point opens the heart's chamber inside the chest and increases emotional intimacy. The Sea of Tranquility also balances the emotions.

Applications for Intercourse: Front-to-front intercourse presses CV 17 naturally as you embrace. When you snuggle, your breast-bones fit together like puzzle pieces, and you feel a heart connection. To open this point and your hearts, place the palms of your hands behind your partner's upper back and hug firmly while you breathe deeply together.

After intercourse, try kissing and sucking the Sea of Tranquility point. After your lips stimulate the point, hug your lover and breathe deeply together in unison as a romantic expression.

For using this point in other love positions, see Embracing Love in Chapter 9 and the Lovemaking Progressions at the end of this chapter.

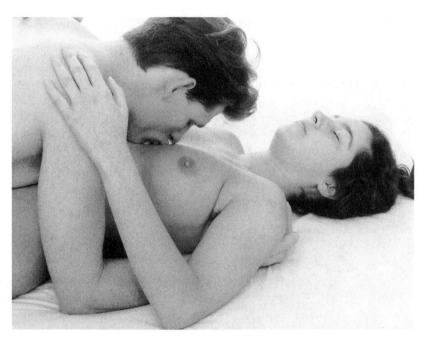

Crooked Bone (CV 2) *and Transverse Bone* (K 11)

Caution: Use both of these points carefully during pregnancy.

Location: CV 2 is on the top edge of the pubic bone, in the center. K 11 is one-half finger-width from the midline on either side, also on the upper border of the pubic bone.

Benefits: Holding these points increases sexual energy and awareness and regulates the sexual-reproductive system.

Applications for Intercourse: All of the front-to-front intercourse postures press these points, opening your sexual energy.

The size differences of couples may mean these points are not getting direct stimulation. In various positions, explore how to adjust your bodies so that your pelvic bones are flush together. Such slight adjustments can greatly heighten your sexual interaction.

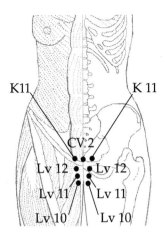

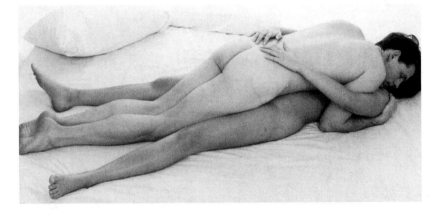

Sex is the "greatest magical force in nature"; an impulse acts in it which suggests the mystery of the One.

—Julius Evola
Magnetic Attraction

Inner Thigh (Lv 10–Lv 12)

Location: On the inside of the upper thigh, close to the inner crease where the thigh joins the trunk of the body.

Benefits: Holding and pressing these points is incredibly sensitive and arousing for lovers. It increases the circulation into the reproductive organs, heightening sensitivity in the genital region.

Applications for Intercourse: These points are stimulated naturally in most intercourse positions. They are particularly important for men, since they trigger life energy into the scrotum.

For using these points to arouse a man, see Chapter 7.

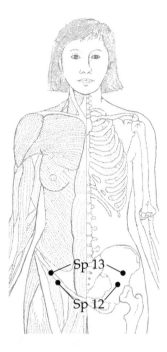

Rushing Door (Sp 12) *and Mansion Cottage* (Sp 13)

Location: In the groin, on the middle of the crease where the leg joins the trunk of the body.

Benefits: Holding these points particularly increases sexual intimacy and enhances sensations in the genitals.

Applications for Intercourse: Apply palm pressure gradually to these points before engaging in intercourse. To open the Rushing Door points and increase the flow of sexual energy into the genitals, hold them for 2 minutes while breathing deeply.

During front-to-front intercourse, grasp hold of your partner's pelvis, bringing the palms of your hands into contact with the base of your partner's hip bone. With your fingers on the sides of your partner's buttocks, rotate your thumbs until they find a thick ropy muscle band in the groin, halfway between the hip bone and the tip of the pubic bone. Holding these points while grasping the pelvis firmly with your hands can be incredibly arousing during intercourse.

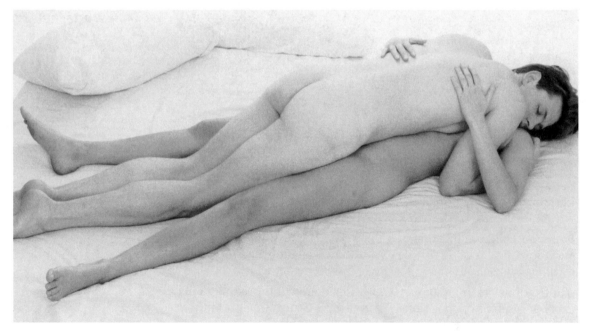

POINTS TO PRESS WITH YOUR HANDS
DURING INTERCOURSE

Select one or two of the following acupressure points to hold during intercourse. The most comfortable points to hold will spontaneously change each time you make love in a different position. When your hand is rotated differently or your body posture or movements vary, your finger pressure applications must also change to stimulate the points effectively. Remember to use natural body mechanics, including leverage and leaning your weight, to hold acupressure points during intercourse.

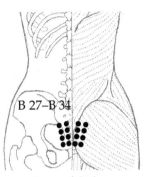

Base of Spine

Sacral Points (B 27–B 34)

Location: On the base of the spine (sacrum), in the hollows of the bone.

Benefits: Steady, firm pressure on these sacral points increases genital pleasure.

Applications for Intercourse: Gradually apply firm pressure to the slight indentations of the sacral bone while making love, which significantly increases sexual pleasure. Using the fingertips of both hands, pull your partner's pelvis close to you. This will strongly stimulate the acupressure points on your pubic bone and enable deeper penetration.

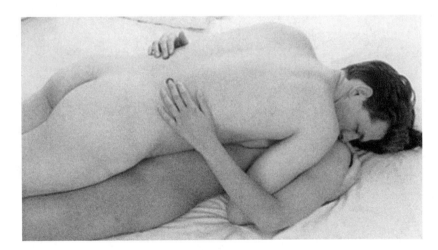

Sexual orgasm can trigger an ecstatic experience. Intercourse does deautomatize somewhat our ordinary reality orientation. It does take us out of ourselves; it is an experience of passionate unity.

—A. M. Greeley
Ecstasy

191

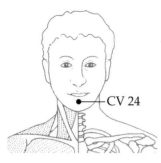

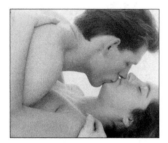

CV 24

Supporting Nourishment (CV 24)

Location: In the indentation midway between the center of your lower lip and your chin.

Benefits: Pressing this point relaxes the facial muscles. In a romantic setting, it can increase intimacy and erotic feelings by heightening awareness of your lips and your sexual energy.

Applications for Intercourse: Touch this point while you are making love, and breathing deeply in sync. Your sexual intimacy may build as you open your partner's lips while doing so.

Kissing this point can deepen your partner's sexual experience. When you are on top of your partner engaging in intercourse, try sucking this point. Communicate how much you want your partner by the intensity of your suction.

Other applications for using this point appear in Embracing Love and A Reconnecting Couple's Routine in Chapter 9.

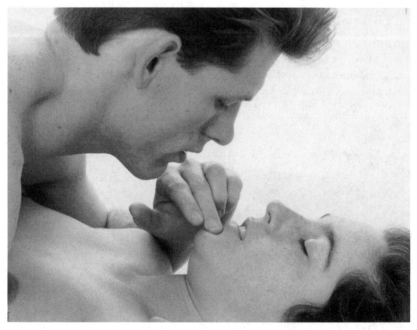

Sea of Vitality (B 23 and B 47)

Caution: Do not press on disintegrating discs or fractured or broken bones. If you have a weak back, a few minutes of stationary light touching instead of pressure can be very healing. See your doctor first if you have any questions or need medical advice.

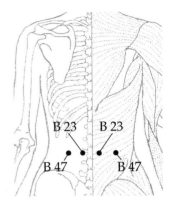

Location: On the lower back (between the second and third lumbar vertebrae), two and four finger-widths away from the spine at waist level, in line with the belly button.

Benefits: Holding this point enhances intimacy and sexual vitality and helps relieve sexual-reproductive problems, including impotence and premature ejaculation.

Applications for Intercourse: During intercourse, place one of your hands over the lower back, positioning your other hand over that hand for support. Firmly squeeze the ropelike muscular cords on both sides of the spine, using your fingertips on one side and the heel of your hand on the other for 1 or 2 minutes.

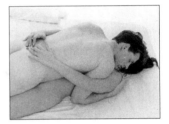

The Sea of Vitality points are powerfully stimulated in Soaring Eagle in Chapter 8 and in the Lovemaking Progressions later in this chapter.

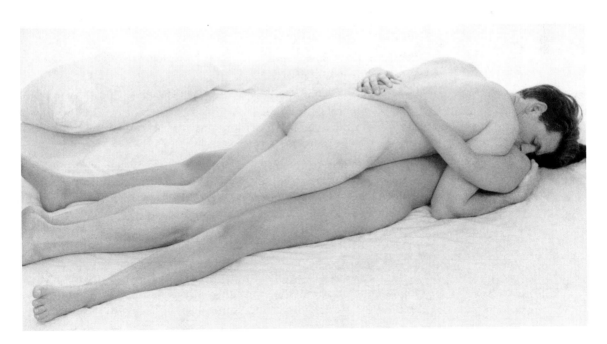

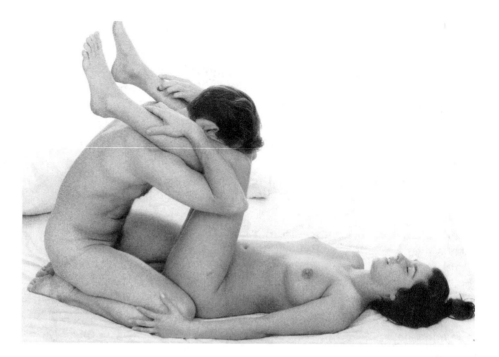

Three Yin Meeting (Sp 6)

Caution: This point nourishes a woman's reproductive system. Do not stimulate it after the seventh month of pregnancy.

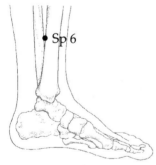

Location: Four finger-widths above the inside anklebone, on the back border of the shinbone.

Benefits: Sp 6 is famous for treating the female sexual-reproductive system, since it connects with the uterus. Holding it regularly develops a nurturing disposition and can bring out the innermost loving qualities in your partner.

Applications for Intercourse: The woman lies on her back, and the man kneels between her feet, putting them up on his shoulders. Holding her ankles, he gently presses 4 finger-widths above the inside of her anklebone. At Sp 6 there is a slight indentation in the bone. If your partner finds the point particularly tender, use light pressure so it doesn't hurt. Relax in a comfortable position, and breathe deeply in sync. Gaze into each other's eyes as your partner lightly caresses your inner thighs up to your sacred organs. When you are both aroused, the man can gently penetrate the vagina, while holding the Three Yin meeting points that connect with the uterus.

Sp 6 is used in the couple's exercise Riding Your Lover in Chapter 8.

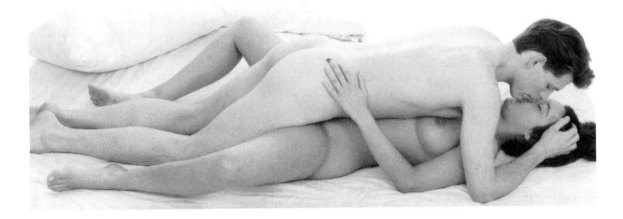

Womb and Vitals (B 48)

Location: One to two finger-widths outside the sacrum (the large bony area at the base of the spine), midway between the top of the hip bone (iliac crest) and the base of the buttocks.

Benefits: As their name indicates, the Womb and Vitals points strongly nurture the sexual-reproductive system. Holding these points on your female partner increases circulation through the pelvis, nourishing her womb and reproductive organs.

Applications for Intercourse: Grasping hold of your partner's "love handles" during intercourse can stimulate B 48 inadvertently. While you are hugging your partner in bed, press these points in the buttocks with your fingertips. Gradually move closer to your partner's body, and press on the outside of your partner's buttocks into the base of the spine at hip level. Since the Womb and Vitals points are located underneath the large buttocks muscles, deeper pressure than your fingers can give is often needed. Try using either the heel of your hands or the knuckles of your fist to apply firm pressure into these points.

The couple's exercise Riding Your Lover in Chapter 8 also stimulates the Womb and Vitals points.

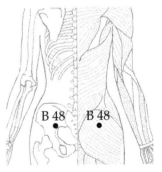

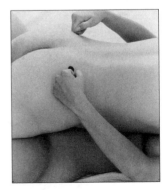

195

LOVE POSITIONS LEADING TO INTERCOURSE

The way you touch your partner and move your body can deepen your intimacy. The more you experiment and play together, the greater your sexual flow becomes.

Womb and Vitals Rock

Certain ways of touching your legs may arouse you to heights that you have rarely experienced before. Simply moving your legs while they are being gently caressed can be an incredible adventure.

Imagine that your legs are the root of your being: strong, soft, and secure. As your partner moves, stretches, and caresses your legs, breathe deeply into their strength and sensuality. Making love is a sacred dance. Enter this dance, opening your mind, body, and spirit to sharing your innermost self with your partner.

Directions

1. Begin with your clothes off. Your partner is lying on his or her back, legs bent, knees up toward the chest. Kneel at your partner's feet, placing your hands on the base of his or her calves. Slowly bring your partner's legs forward and slide your knees underneath your partner's buttocks.

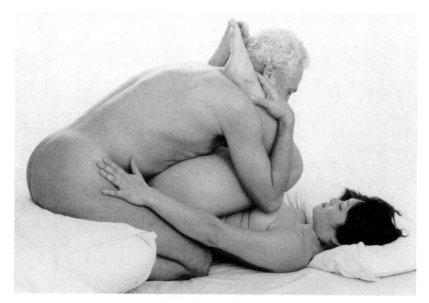

As the lead and response of good dancers appears to be almost simultaneous, as if they were a single entity, there comes a moment when more intimate sexual contact occurs with an extraordinary mutuality. The man does not lead and the woman follow; the man-and-woman relationship acts of itself. His "advance" and her "response" seems to be in the same moment.

—Alan Watts
Nature, Man, and Woman

2. Rock the knees slowly forward and backward, bringing them into your partner's chest.

3. Place your partner's feet onto the center of your chest. Gradually lean forward, slowly rocking your body back and forth.

4. Gradually bring your partner's feet in toward his or her sit bones.

5. With your partner's legs spread apart, gradually lean your chest toward him or her as you firmly hug the legs. Slowly rock your partner's legs forward and backward, maintaining eye contact. Gently touch and kiss your partner in this intimate position.

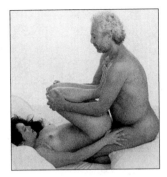

Suggestions

Interlace your fingers with your partner's, maintaining eye contact as you extend your partner's arms up and over his or her head.

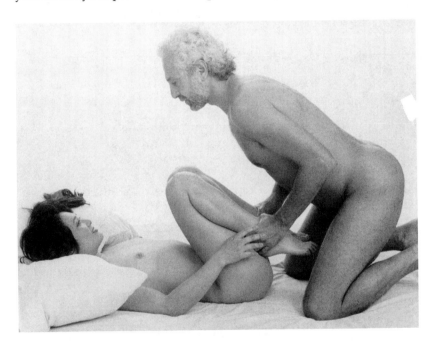

Finding the most suitable position for both partners is vitally important. It can take ten or more encounters before they become used to one another's bodies—and even then, if they continue to experiment, they may discover still better and better positions.

—Jolan Chang
The Tao of Love and Sex

197

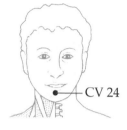

CV 24

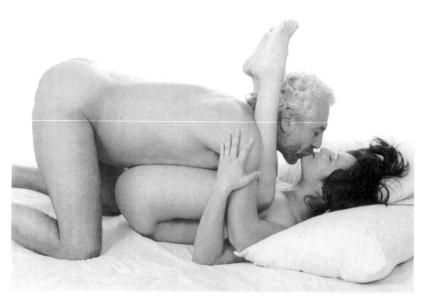

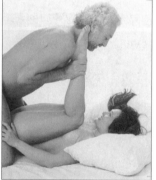

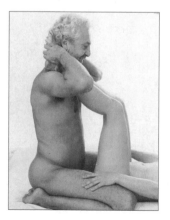

Variations

Place your partner's feet on your shoulders, and slowly rock your upper body back and forth, holding your partner's knees. Feel free to lean all the way back, stretching your partner's legs.

In the same position, with your partner's calves on your shoulders, slowly lean forward, bringing your chests together. If you are stretched out enough, you may be able to kiss. After enjoying your partner's lips, try kissing the acupressure point between the lower lip and the chin (CV 24). Sucking this point firmly can be quite arousing.

Grasp hold of your partner's Achilles tendon, with your thumbs inside and your fingers outside the ankle. Slowly bring the feet forward, gently stretching the backs of your partner's legs. Do this gradually and carefully, encouraging your partner to give you feedback on how far to stretch.

Rest your partner's ankles on your shoulders. Reach your arms up and over to massage your partner's feet. Massage the bottoms of your partner's feet with your fingertips, while the heels of your hands massage the tops. Then rake your fingertips between the bones on the tops of the feet. Continue to glide your fingertips lightly from the tops of the feet over the inside of your partner's legs toward the genitals—the slower and gentler the better.

The Vitality Saver

Here's a technique for allowing men to ejaculate without feeling sleepy and tired afterward. Simply continue in the same positions previously described.

The woman's heels are on the man's shoulders. He leans forward, resting his elbows beside her shoulders. When it feels right, he slowly enters her vagina by tilting his pelvis toward her. As they strongly embrace each other, either partner can hold the man's Inner Meeting (CV 1) point between the anus and genitals.

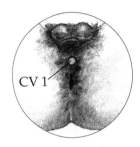

To press this CV 1 point during intercourse, reach around the buttocks with one hand and feel for an indentation exactly halfway between the scrotum and anus. Deep pressure must be applied in order to feel this small, hollow space. Before and during ejaculation, press this point firmly into the indentation to obtain the full benefits. Holding this point focuses a man's awareness and can increase his pleasure during orgasm.

Usually people must practice using this point a few times before they learn the proper timing, location, and angle of pressure. If the point is not pressed firmly enough or in the right location, the man may find his urine to be cloudy or especially bubbly after ejaculating, indicating that semen moved into the bladder and mixed with the urine. This backup into the bladder is not dangerous and has no side effects. Holding the point correctly blocks the semen from going through the penis and into the bladder.

As you hold this point, you will feel throbbing pulsations from the prostate gland. The pressure of your finger is blocking the flow

In sexual intercourse,

semen must be

regarded as a most

precious substance.

By saving it,

a man protects

his very life.

—Peng-tze
Secrets of the Jade Bedroom

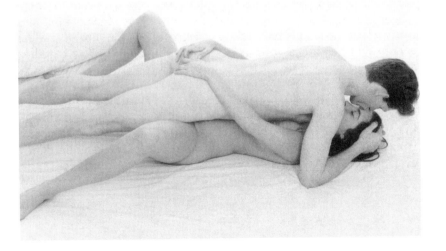

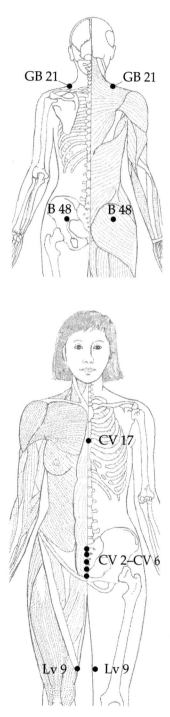

of semen, preventing it from being released, and channeling it into the prostate, from which it will be recycled into the bloodstream. The ejaculation thus occurs internally. Most of the essence is not lost, although small amounts of semen can be found in the clear fluid that leaks out of the penis. But most of the nutrients from the semen are recycled back into the body.

Pressing CV 1 correctly can rechannel a man's energy, heighten his vitality, and enable him to be awake and present with his partner after an orgasm. Instead of dozing off to sleep, he can actively share intimacy. Women absolutely love the results of this point; men find it rewarding, satisfying, and refreshing. When a man can be fully intimate with his partner, a sexual relationship takes on a new life.

Acupressure Points

Point	Name	Location
B 48	*Womb and Vitals*	In the buttocks
GB 21	*Shoulder Well*	On the tops of the shoulders
CV 2–CV 6	*Sea of Intimacy*	In the lower abdomen
CV 17	*Sea of Tranquility*	In the center of the breastbone
LV 9	*Joy of Living*	On the inside of the thighs
CV 1	*Inner Meeting*	Between the rectum and genitals

Benefits: This advanced couple's exercise strongly benefits the lower back, legs, and pelvis. In acupressure terms, it opens the bladder and kidney meridians. It stretches the sciatic or "life" nerve, the largest nerve in the body. Stretching it regularly enables a couple to live a longer life together. Once you and your partner are stretched out and ready, these variations may release a tremendous amount of healing energy that heightens your ability to deeply connect, play together, and make love.

Pressing CV 1 several seconds prior to and during a man's orgasm often enhances his pleasure and increases the duration of his orgasm. Since a man knows when he is about to ejaculate, it is natural for him to hold the point on himself. When his partner learns where the point is located and how to hold it, however, the pleasure is heightened even more.

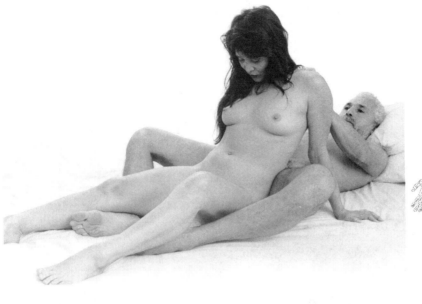

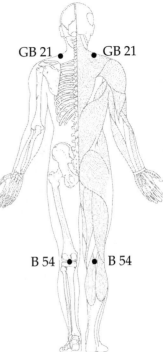

A LOVING LOUNGE CHAIR

This routine culminates in front-to-back intercourse. The instructions are directed to the male partner in a heterosexual relationship, but they can be adapted for lovers of any persuasion.

Directions

1. Lie on your back, with your head resting on a pillow and your legs spread wide open. Your partner, facing away from you, sits between your thighs. As you breathe deeply together, your bodies relax into each other. Imagine you are in a romantic environment together, outside in the sun.

2. Your partner's upper body weight is supported with her arms as she comfortably leans back.

3. Bend your legs, bringing your inner anklebones underneath the center of the crease behind your lover's knees, pressing acupressure point B 54.

4. Bring your hands to your partner's shoulders (GB 21). Slowly and firmly knead out any shoulder tension.

While making love, neither of you should stop touching each other with your hands, until you are both tired and ready to go to sleep.

—Jolan Chang
The Tao of Love and Sex

201

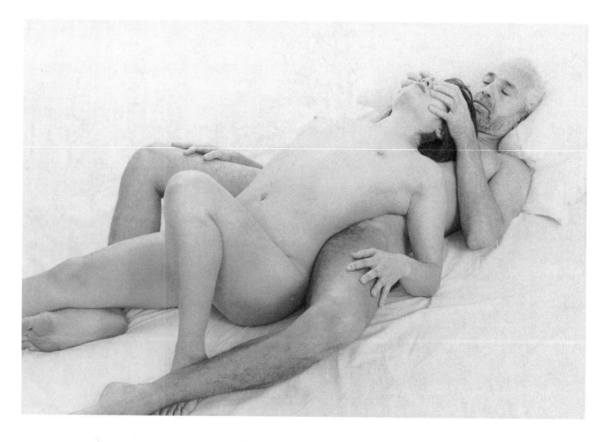

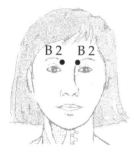

5. After a minute or two, invite her to lie down comfortably, resting the back of her head on the center of your body.

6. Place your index and middle fingertips on the inside corners of her upper eye sockets (B 2), close to the bridge of the nose. Then gently massage her scalp and face, including the temples, jaws, and ears.

Suggestions

Breathe deeply together into your bellies, letting them swell like balloons on the inhalation, and letting yourselves go on the exhalation. After you inhale deeply, make a long releasing "ahhhh" sound, letting go of any internalized stress. Keep your eyes closed as you and your partner make this sound together. Increase the intensity of the volume, and enjoy listening to its healing vibrations.

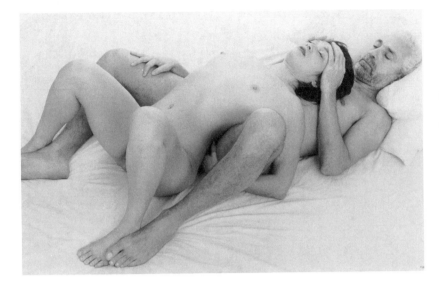

Advanced Variations

- Your lover lies on her back between your legs. Her feet are flat on the floor, close to her buttocks and spread a shoulder-width apart. Place the bottoms of your feet gently on top of her thighs. As her pelvis begins to rise, firmly push the balls of your feet forward against her thighs. Close your eyes and continue moving your pelvis up and down together for a minute or two. This pelvic movement gently stretches the thighs, pelvis, and lower back.

- Both you and your partner bend your legs, placing your feet flat on the floor. Your partner above you reaches around the outside of your thighs to explore the area between your legs. Breathe deeply into your belly, giving her plenty of time to find the point between your rectum and genitals (CV 1). While she firmly holds this potent point, massage her head or shoulders, gradually giving compression with the heels of your hands as you slowly knead. Your partner gently fondles the intimate areas between your legs.

When the same inner sight exists in you as in another, you are drawn to be companions. When a man feels in himself the inmost nature of a woman, he is drawn to her sexually. When a woman feels the masculine self of a man within her, she wants him physically in her.

—John Moyne
and Coleman Barks
Open Secret, Versions of Rumi

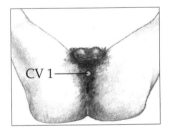

203

Desire smiles at the Woman in Love, tickles her with her toes, races her from shore to shore. Desire squeezes the nipples of the Woman in Love, and molds her breasts, kisses her with a probing demand, a wanting that will not be stilled. Desire pulls the Woman in Love into the sand and reaches inside her suit, inside her body, pushing her want forward. The Woman in Love pushes back to meet her, to match her, to open to this mating so sunwrapped, thrust upon her, so longed-for and feared and revered. Coming, she loses contact with all but the radiating sensations centered in her groin, in her ass. . . . She burrows into her lover's shoulder, into her lover's breast.

—Tee Corinne
"Dreams of the Woman
Who Loved Sex"

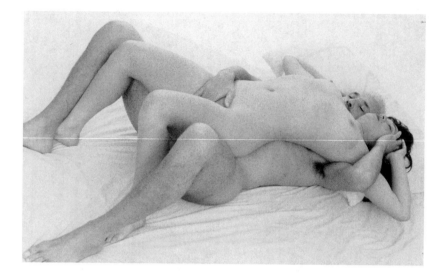

The following variations involve more body weight and require greater flexibility.

• If your partner's back is strong and limber, she can reach up and back to join hands with you. Once you both have a good grasp of each other's wrists or hands, gradually straighten your arms and stretch your partner way up onto your chest so that her hands hang back over your shoulders.

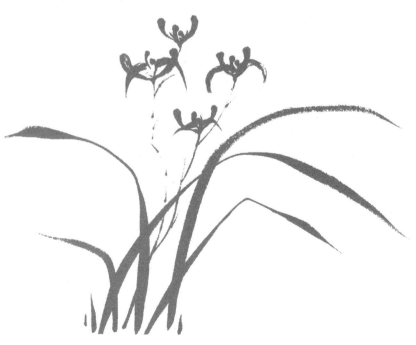

- Readjust your bodies in this position, placing your temples together. Both of you hold your palms firmly against each other's outer ears, blocking out any sound. Close your eyes. Take a deep breath together, and exhale as you make an "ong" sound. Try harmonizing your sound a few more times.

- Place your hands over her breasts, taking time to enjoy the connection. Feel for her nipples and stimulate St 17. Slowly roll the nipples between your thumb and fingertips as you breathe deeply. Turn your head toward your partner, kissing, licking, and gently nibbling her ear.

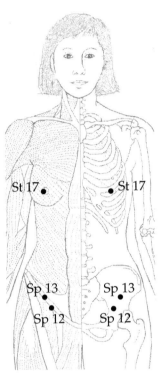

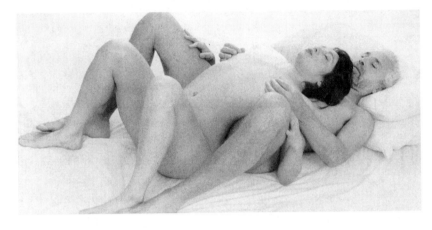

- **Penetration from the Back:** Slowly roll onto your sides into a spooning position. Caress your partner's groin, vaginal lips, and eventually her clitoris. When your penis is hard and she is aroused, gently penetrate her from behind. Hold her groin points (Sp 12, Sp 13) with your fingertips as you grasp and move her hips erotically back and forth.

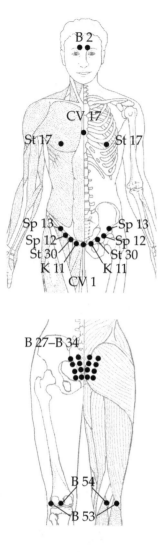

Acupressure Points

Point	Name	Location
B 2	*Drilling Bamboo*	In an indentation of the upper eye socket at the inside of the eyebrow
CV 17	*Sea of Tranquility*	On the center of the breastbone, four finger-widths up from the base of the breastbone
St 17	*Center of the Breast*	On the center of the nipple
K 11	*Transverse Bone*	One-half inch from the midline of the pubic bone
St 30	*Energy Rushing*	On the outer tips of the pubic bone
Sp 12	*Rushing Door*	Between the hip and pubic bone, in the center of the groin
Sp 13	*Mansion Cottage*	
B 27–B 34	*Sacral Points*	At the base of the spine, directly above the tailbone
B 53	*Active Command*	In the outer edge of the crease behind the knee
B 54	*Commanding Middle*	In the center of the crease in back of the knee
CV 1	*Inner Meeting*	In the hollow midway between the anus and genitals

Benefits: This couple's posture can open a new way for making contact with each other. Lying back-to-front opens up the diaphragm and chest for deeper breathing. It also opens the heart cavity, abdomen, and pelvis. The gentle stretching and the stimulation of the points directs healing energy into the reproductive organs.

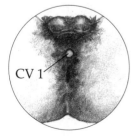

LOVEMAKING PROGRESSIONS

Taking time to explore each other and discover new ways to touch and embrace is important in a love relationship. Before you engage in intercourse, take time to massage each other, stretch your bodies, breathe together, touch every part of each other's bodies, and enjoy gazing into each other's eyes.

This routine takes you through an intimate transformation for making love. Begin by standing close to each other, face to face.

Mutual Massage

While one partner massages the shoulders and the neck, the other massages the lower back and firmly kneads the buttocks muscles. Then switch; if you were massaging the lower back, now massage the shoulders and the neck. If you find it more relaxing to be entirely receptive while your partner massages you for a few minutes, alternate massage with your partner.

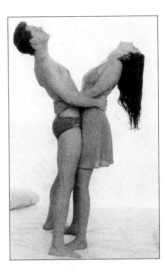

Couple's Stretching

Support your lower backs by embracing each other around the waist. With your knees slightly bent, pelvis to pelvis, slowly tilt your heads backward, lifting your chests up and out as you inhale together. Exhale, and firmly hug your partner. Repeat this breathing exercise a few more times. As you inhale and arch back, straighten your arms and curve your fingers to hook into your partner's lower back muscles. As you exhale and come close, enjoy kissing your partner on the lips.

Full-Body Hug-You Pressure

Hug your partner firmly, wrapping your arms around each other. Make full-body contact with your feet, thighs, pelvises, bellies, and chests. Lift your chins up, creating a powerful connection with the front of your throats together. As you continue to hug, use your arm muscles to bring your partner's body into you. Then slowly but firmly knead the muscles of your partner's back, from the buttocks all the way up through the neck.

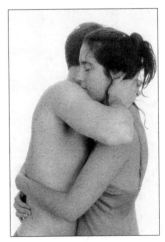

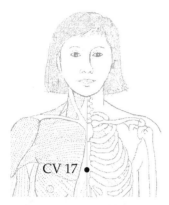

CV 17 •

Full-Heart Hug

Embrace your partner, wrapping your arms around him or her and breathing deeply into your hearts. In this position, line up your breastbones to press on the Sea of Tranquility (CV 17). If one of you is much taller than the other, the taller of you might want to bend your knees and tilt the pelvis forward, if it brings your bodies closer. Once your bodies fit together, squeeze your partner firmly. In a gentle but passionate way, use your teeth to gnaw as well as suck on your partner's shoulder, neck, and earlobes. Enjoy kissing on the lips.

Help your partner lie down comfortably on his or her back, with knees bent, feet flat on the carpet or bed.

Drinking the Love

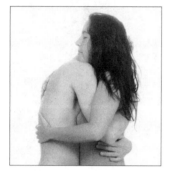

With your partner's head on a pillow, hands out to the sides, kneel at your partner's feet and place your hands on his or her knees. Gracefully lean forward, slowly pushing your partner's knees toward his or her armpits. (Due to the structure of the pelvis, women tend to be more flexible than men in this posture.) Lift your partner's feet upward as you slowly lean forward, bringing your shoulders into the back crease of your partner's knees. With your arms embracing your partner's thighs, slowly rock his or her legs back and forth as you breathe deeply together.

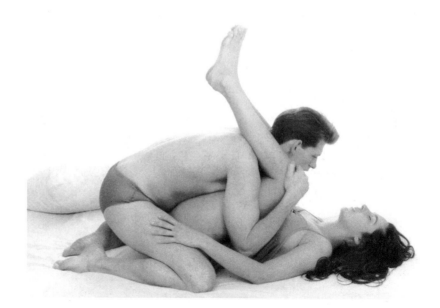

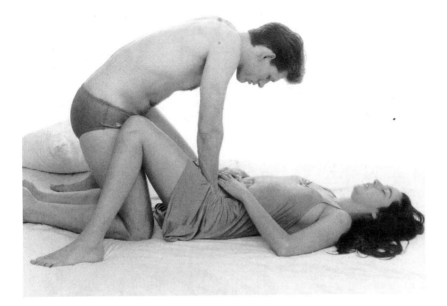

Suggestions

As the partner on top slowly shifts his or her weight downward and/or forward, ask the other partner for feedback about how the stretch feels.

If the partner on the bottom gets a groin cramp, simply bring his or her legs outward and slowly apply palm pressure on the crease where the leg joins the trunk of the body. Gradually lean your upper-body weight on the ropelike cord that runs from the base of the hip bone to the tip of the pubic bone. A couple of minutes of palm pressure on these points in the groin (Sp 12 and Sp 13) with long deep belly-breathing will relieve the cramping.

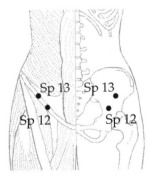

The Heart's Pleasure

Readjust your bodies to find a position that is mutually comfortable to maintain eye contact. Hold your partner in this position, and begin long, deep breathing together, inhaling and exhaling at the same time. Slowly lower the center of your chest comfortably onto your partner's genitals. Close your eyes, breathe deeply together, and feel the connection.

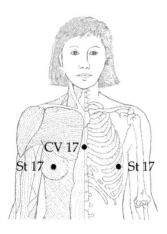

Variations

The partner on top can take an active role to initiate some of the following lovemaking activities:

- **Kissing the Sea of Tranquility:** Reach around from the outside of your partner's body to hold the shoulders as you lean forward to kiss and apply suction to the center of his or her breastbone (CV 17).

    Instead of holding your partner's shoulders or knees, place your hands on point St 17, located on your partner's nipples. Using your thumbs and index fingers, slowly roll the nipples back and forth between your fingertips. Begin gently, gradually increasing the firmness of the roll. Breathe in sync with the depth and intensity of your partner's breath. After a while you may feel inclined to suck the nipples.

I open my heart at daybreak; a maiden plucks me and kisses me and puts me to her breast. I am the abode of happiness and the source of joy.

—Kahlil Gibran
A Tear and a Smile

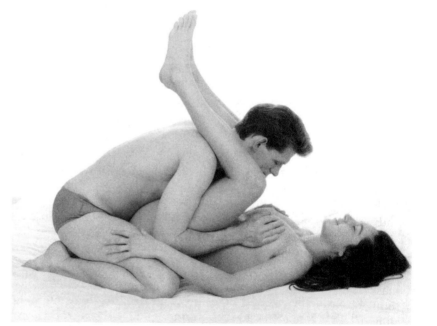

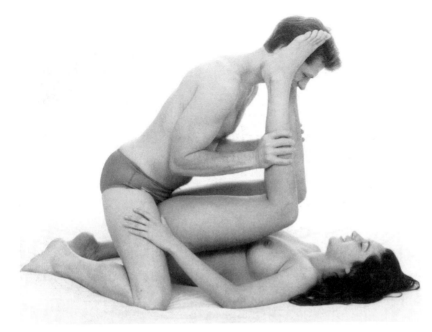

Sex is the joy of discovery and the beauty of shared pleasure. Sex is part of the life force. The giving and receiving of sexual energy is our birthright. Sexual pleasure, in its biggest meaning, is a life energy, a healing force.

—Joan Nelson
"Lighting Candles"

- **Changing the Diaper:** For this variation, remove the pillow. If your partner is limber, grasp hold of your partner's ankles, slowly bringing the feet up and over the body. Scoot your knees underneath your partner's lower back or buttocks. As you slowly lower your partner's legs toward you, the weight of his or her body on your knees applies acupressure to a number of points in the lower back and pelvic area. Slowly rock your partner's legs forward and backward. Continue to reposition your knees for maximum comfort and release.

- **Taking Your Time:** Bend your partner's legs, bringing his or her knees toward the armpits. Then place his or her feet on the tops of your shoulders with the arches against the side of your neck. Now massage your partner's feet, ankles, and buttocks. Then use your thumbs to gently press the soft tissue area between the anus and the sit bones. Massaging this area with your thumbs very slowly can be quite pleasurable, especially to an athletic person.

    Place your hands on the back of your partner's thighs, and very slowly push the legs forward and apart. Let your head relax downward, kissing, sucking, and licking what's before you. Breathe deeply and take your time.

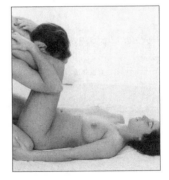

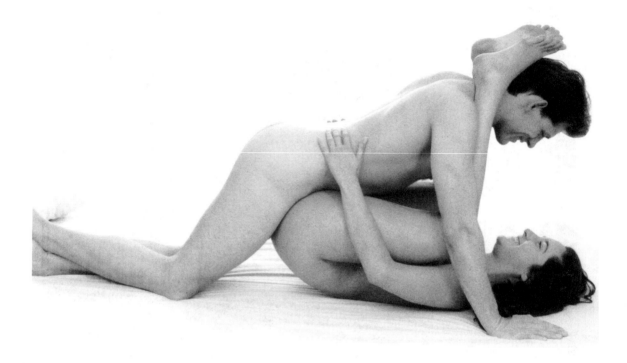

Draw back the shaft

And you miss it.

Raise the arrow head,

And you overshoot it.

Aim below the navel,

And you enter it.

—Yu Hsien Ku
Chen Wen-Cheng

• **Making Love in a Capsule:** With your partner's legs spread apart, rest his or her feet over your shoulders and kneel between the thighs. Place the palms of your hands on the floor above your partner's shoulders, slowly bringing your body forward. Gradually lower your pelvis until you have gentle contact with your partner's genitals. Breathe deeply, gaze into your partner's eyes, and enjoy touching each other. When you are both completely aroused, engage in intercourse.

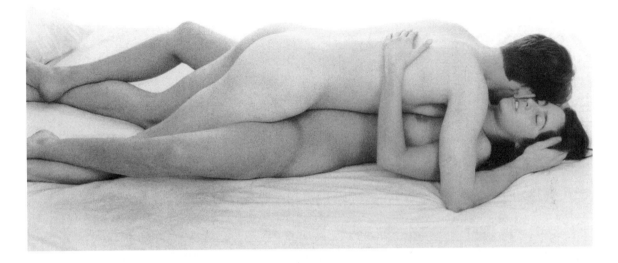

Slowly lower your upper body until you are lying with your lover breast to breast, heart to heart. Rest your elbows on the floor, placing your fingers up on top of your partner's head. With his or her eyes closed, use the heels of your hands to firmly press the opening of your partner's ears, blocking out any sound.

At the same time, your partner can wrap his or her arms around your lower back. Your partner's feet can stroke the length of your calf muscles, gradually gliding back down to connect with your feet.

- **During intercourse,** kiss each other on the lips, cheeks, eyes, temples, ears, throat, breasts—all over, until you are thoroughly intoxicated with your partner's energy. Then passionately wrap your bodies close together, embracing in another full-body hug. Gently move your pelvis back and forth, stopping before he reaches his climax to prolong intercourse. The more you practice this strategy for extending intercourse, the longer you will be able to make love. Breathe deeply together, letting your bodies slide passionately back and forth, moving together, meshing together, eventually melting into one.

The true joy of loving is an ecstasy of two bodies and souls mingling and uniting in poetry.

—Jolan Chang
The Tao of Love and Sex

213

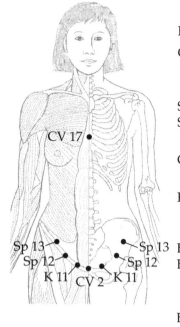

Acupressure Points

Point	Name	Location
CV 17	*Sea of Tranquility*	On the center of the breastbone, four finger-widths up from the base of the bone
Sp 12 Sp 13	*Rushing Door* *Mansion Cottage*	In the groin, on the middle of the crease where the leg joins the trunk of the body
CV 2	*Crooked Bone*	On the top edge of the pubic bone in the center
K 11	*Transverse Bone*	One-half finger-width from the midline, on the upper border of the pubic bone
B 23 B 47	*Sea of Vitality*	On the lower back, 2 and 4 finger-widths away from the spine at waist level, in line with the belly button
B 27–B 34	*Sacral Points*	On the base of the spine (sacrum), in the hollows of the bone
B 51	*Prosperous Gate*	On the center of the back of the thigh

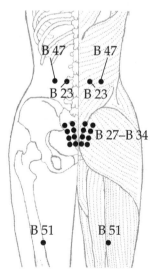

If it is true that the "Spirit feels nothing except with the help of the body," it is also true that the body is called upon, is appointed to bring the spirit into the world, to be delivered of it. There can be no great couple without strong sexuality, nor can there be one that has not learned to fetch it in and master it.

—Suzanne Lilar
"The Sacred Dimension"

Chapter 11

THAI MASSAGE AND ADVANCED COUPLE WORK

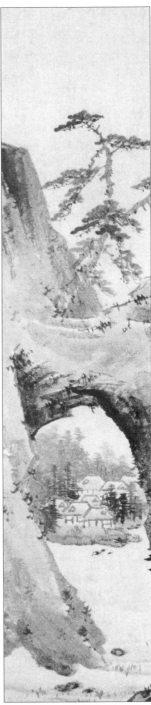

This chapter presents acupressure techniques, Thai massage, and the Oriental bodywork method called shiatsu. Thai massage involves a dynamic series of stretches for increased flexibility and deep relaxation. Shiatsu uses body weight to apply firm pressure gradually into your partner's body.

In this chapter you will learn two multistep routines for giving your partner intimate mutual care. They will increase the circulation of blood and the flow of energy through the groin, pelvis, and legs. Practicing these dynamic bodywork and stretching routines in couples often releases a great deal of erotic, sexual energy.

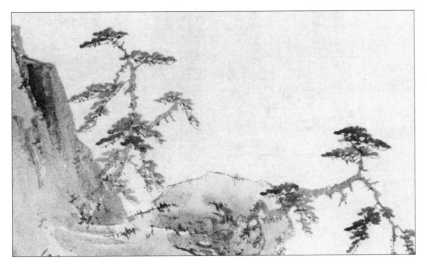

STRETCHES FOR LOVERS

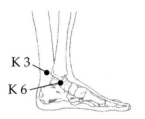

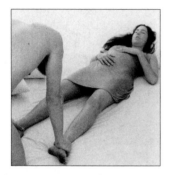

Have your partner lie comfortably on his or her back on a carpeted floor or on top of a bed. Sit at your partner's feet and place your fingertips on the tops of the feet and your thumbs on the arches. Slowly massage your partner's feet as you take full, deep breaths to collect your energy. Lean forward, and squeeze both your fingers and thumbs together, grasping the whole foot. Start at the lower portion of the arch, pressing with your thumb near the heel. Inch by inch, press up the arch as you squeeze with your whole hand.

Grasping all of the toes, lean forward and move the tops of your partner's feet up toward the knees and outward. This movement stretches the Achilles tendon and the calf muscles. It also gently opens the upper leg.

Place the palms of your hands on the arch and lean forward again. Then use your thumbs to press Bigger Stream (K 3) and Joyful Sleep (K 6), located in the soft area between the inner anklebone and the heel. These points benefit the sexual-reproductive system. If they are sore, be sure to press them gently.

Slowly walk your palms up your partner's legs, pressing gently on the calves and knees. Continue all the way up the thighs to tantalize the groin. Place the heel of your hand on the Rushing Door and Mansion Cottage points (Sp 12 and Sp 13), in the groin between your partner's hip bone and pubic bone. Slowly lean the weight of your chest over your hands. Ask your partner to breathe into his or her belly for at least 1 minute, giving firm, steady pressure.

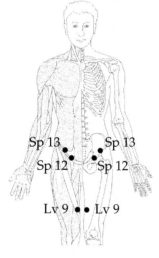

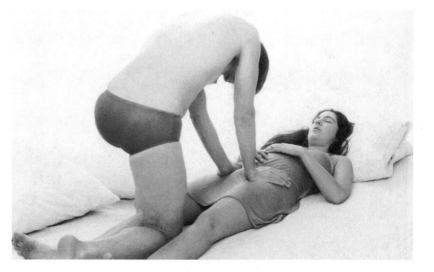

Walk your hands down the leg to the knees, then cup your hands and make circular movements on the kneecaps. Again, ask your partner to breathe deeply into his or her belly. Then continue to caress your partner's legs, down the calves and the lower portion of the legs, returning to the feet. Now, give your partner a wonderful foot massage on both feet at the same time.

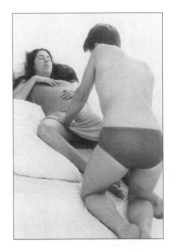

The following five steps should be done on one leg and then on the other.

1. **Caress the Inner Leg:** Place both of your hands on one leg (one hand behind the knee and the other at the foot). Bend the leg outward so the thigh is at a right angle to the lower leg. Place a pillow underneath the bent knee for support. With one hand on the foot, the other on the inner thigh, slowly lean your upper body weight into your palms to apply firm pressure. Each time you palm the thigh, move to a different spot. Fondle up the leg, close to where it attaches near the pubic bone. Meanwhile, move your lower hand gently on the calf. Continue to use palm pressure, walking your hands to different parts of the leg. Then place both hands on the inside of the upper leg, giving firm pressure to the thigh muscles with the heels of your hands.

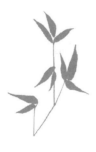

Where your hands have been, I am yours, and your hands

have been everywhere. Your words enter my soil like rain.

Your memory. Oh love, your memory takes me suddenly,

wrenches me from this world into a fairy tale where

I am loved the way I always wanted to be.

—Tee Corinne
"Dreams of the Woman Who Loved Sex"

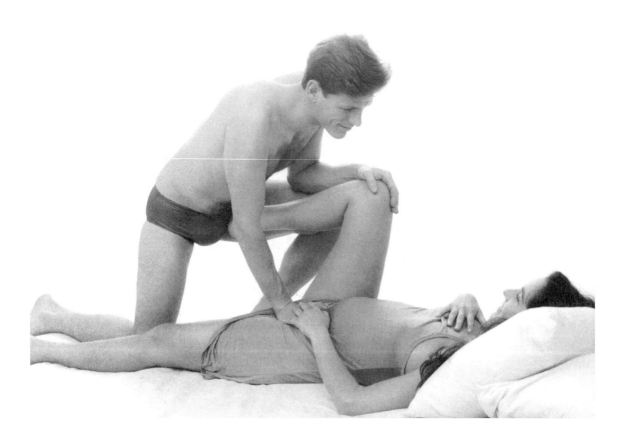

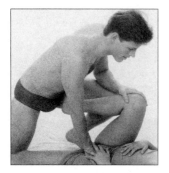

2. **Energize the Thigh:** Lift the leg you just worked on, bringing the knee upward. Place your partner's foot in your groin. Put your outer hand on your partner's knee. Use your other hand to lovingly press and caress your partner's opposite thigh and groin area. Gradually lean into the groin, gently stretching the leg that is bent. Ask your partner to breathe deeply into the stretch and into any feelings that arise.

3. **Stretch the Hamstrings:** Place your partner's foot on your shoulder. Use the palms of both hands to press behind the hamstrings on the back of your partner's thigh. Gently lean some of your weight to apply pressure, stretching your partner's lower back and leg muscles. This stretch also benefits the knee. Be sure to cover the entire back of the thigh, from the sit bone all the way up to the knee crease. Press inward by leaning your weight toward your partner for a few seconds, then fondle and slide to a new area on the back of the thigh.

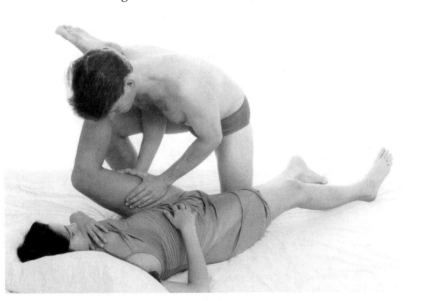

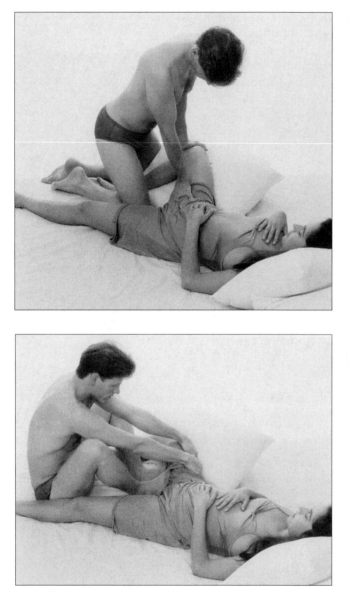

4. **Tantalize the Inner Thigh:** With your partner's leg bent, simply let the knee fall outward. Support your partner's leg by holding the outside of the thigh with your outer hand or by placing a couple of pillows under the outer thigh of the bent leg. Use your other hand to press and caress the inner thigh. You will find a large, thick ropy muscle on the inside of the thigh. Place the heel of your hand underneath this tight muscle, and gradually lean into the center mass of the thigh, pressing inward and upward. With utmost sensitivity and love, focus your attention on the area close to your partner's genitals. This move releases the inside of the leg and often opens up erotic energy in the genital area.

5. **"Juice" the Thigh:** With the leg bent outward, sit between your partner's legs. Place the balls of your feet on the inner thigh. Hook your fingertips over your partner's thigh and slowly lean back. One hand follows the other, covering the front of the thigh. Then bring your partner's foot over your ankle and continue pulling the leg into the balls of your feet. This creates a powerful compression for releasing the muscles in your partner's inner thighs. Change the position of both your feet and your hands to cover various areas of the thigh.

After completing these steps, repeat them on your partner's other leg. Then do the following techniques on both legs.

6. **The Hoover Maneuver:** Raise your partner's legs, forming a right angle with the trunk of his or her body. Instruct your partner to place palms on knees, keeping the elbows straight. Stand to one side of your partner with one foot forward. Grasp both of your partner's ankles while you slowly push the feet above his or her head, bringing the buttocks off the ground. Slowly apply this stretch three or four times.

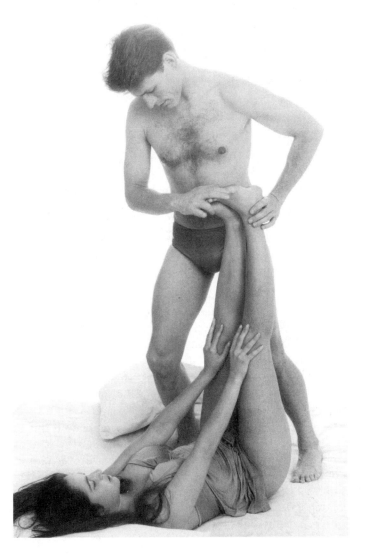

Be a lover as they are, that you come to know your Beloved. Be faithful that you may know Faith. The other parts of the universe did not accept the next responsibility of love as you can. They were afraid they might make a mistake with it, the inspired knowing that springs from being in love.

—Rumi
Open Secret

221

Trust allows you to laugh. You can just as easily laugh and play while you grow as become serious and overwhelmed. Spiritual partners can laugh at the richness and the beauty and the playfulness of the Universe. They enjoy each other. They see the frustrations of the wants of the personality for what they are, learnings, sometimes great learnings, for the soul.

—Gary Zukav
Seat of the Soul

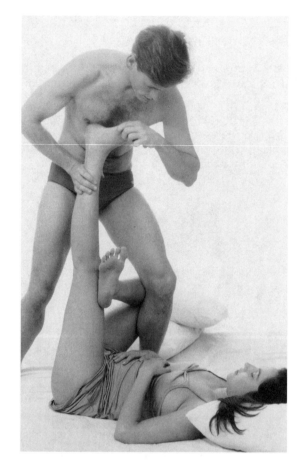

7. **Straddle the Fore Stretch:** Stand, holding one of your partner's legs against your chest. Then cross the foot of your partner's other leg in front of the upright knee. Straddle the out-extended knee. With one hand on the heel and the other hand on the ball of the foot, slowly stretch the leg over your partner's head. This stretches the sciatic nerve, which according to yoga therapy enables you to live a long life.

Make sure that you perform all the movements in this exercise very slowly. After several stretches, slowly let the leg that was stretched come down, and bring the other leg upward. Then cross the other leg with the outside of the foot on the thigh and repeat this exercise by stepping over the out-extended knee. Slowly bring the extended foot up and gradually toward your partner's head. Again, be sure to make the movements slow.

8. **Fondle the Fore Stretch:** Depending on your size, you can kneel or stand with one foot in front of the other, whichever you find more comfortable. Hold the ankle and the knee of your partner's bent leg as you support his or her upright leg with your shoulder. Lean forward as you fondle the inner thigh of the bent leg. After touching all parts of your partner's thigh, switch legs and repeat both this step and Straddle the Fore Stretch on the other side.

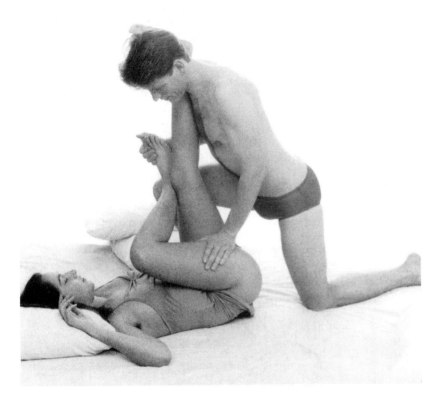

The minute I heard my first love story, I started looking for you, not knowing how blind that was. Lovers don't finally meet somewhere. They're in each other all along.

—John Moyne
and Coleman Barks
Open Secret, Versions of Rumi

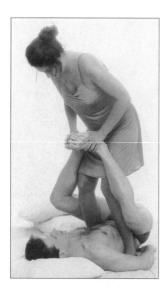

9. **The Froggy Stretch:** With your hands on both ankles, slowly stretch your partner's legs upward over his or her head. Then separate the legs about two feet apart and again gently stretch them over the head. With your partner's arms extended out from his or her body, step over your partner's thighs to stand beside the waist.

Gradually stretch the legs forward, bringing the feet over your partner's head. Repeat this three times. Then bring the bottoms of your partner's feet together as the knees fall outward. While you hold the feet together, slowly bring them down toward your partner's face. Also repeat this stretch three times.

10. **Knees to Chest:** Bend your partner's legs, placing your hands on the outside of his or her knees as you kneel on one knee. Ask your partner to inhale deeply. As your partner exhales, slowly lean your body weight into the knees, bringing them down toward the chest. Release the pressure as your partner inhales, leaning into the stretch as he or she exhales. This exercise relieves a tired, aching lower back. Kneeling on one knee, place your hands below your partner's knees, rocking them back and forth toward the chest. Ask your partner to inhale as you bring his or her knees up toward you. As the knees are pressed toward your partner's chest, exhale. This benefits the lower back and opens up the pelvis and groin.

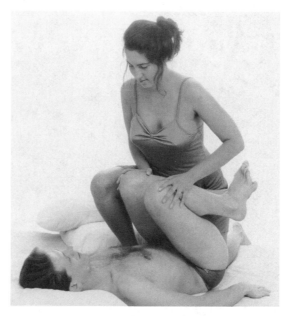

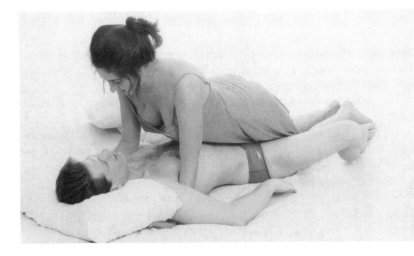

11. **An Exotic Embrace:** Bring your partner's legs out and apart as you kneel between them. Slowly glide your hands over the sides of your partner's body. Slowly lower your pelvis toward your partner. Gradually place your chests together, wrapping your arms around each other in a full-body embrace. Feel free simply to relax into each other or passionately kiss and make love.

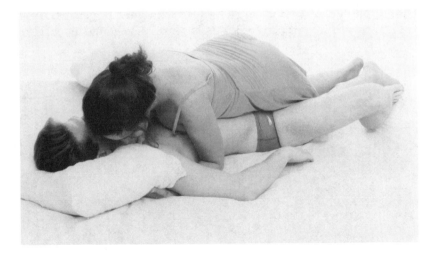

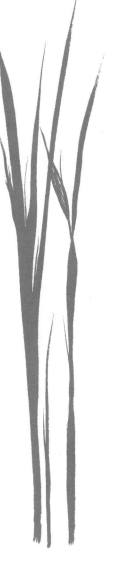

225

THAI BACK MASSAGE

This Thai leg and lower back acupressure massage, performed on a person lying down, is a wonderful stretch routine for relieving general stress, back spasms, and stiffness.

The person to receive the massage should lie down on his or her stomach with legs spread. Position yourself at your partner's heels, and gradually apply firm palm and finger pressure on his or her ankles, heels, Achilles tendons, and feet bottoms. Lean your body, and squeeze your hands into these areas of your partner. Then sensually glide your hands up and down the legs.

Slowly walk the palms of your hands up the back of the thighs, being careful not to apply a great deal of pressure behind the knee. To work on the buttocks, turn your hands inward with your fingertips pointing toward each other. As you lean forward, use the heels of your hands to press deep into the gluteus muscles of the buttocks. Firmly knead the buttocks muscles. As you lean forward, give these muscles extra compression, as if you were kneading dough. You can also knead the lower back muscles in this way. Fit the heels of your hands into the small of the back with your fingertips pointing toward each other, giving firm compression to any tight back muscles.

Slowly glide your fingertips lightly down your partner's thighs and the backs of the knees and calves, all the way down to his or her feet. Lightly caress your partner's legs with your fingertips. Apply more pressure if your partner is overly sensitive to gentle touch.

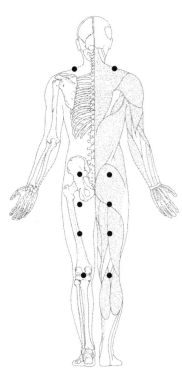

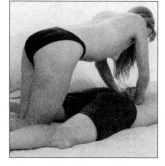

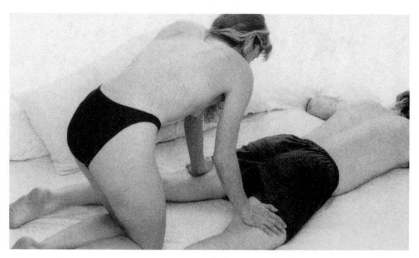

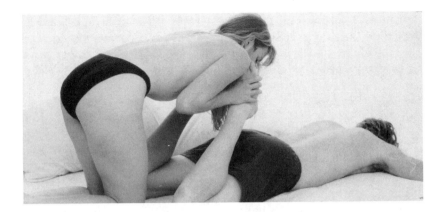

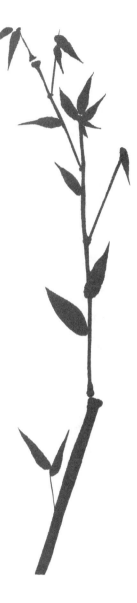

1. **Quad Stretches:** Placing your hands underneath your partner's feet, slowly bend the legs, bringing the feet up toward the buttocks. Gently but firmly stretch the legs. Ask your partner how much pressure he or she needs to make the stretch enjoyable.

2. **Triangle Leg Stretch and Lift:** Place one foot behind the knee crease of the other leg. Very slowly lean the foot that is upward in toward your partner's buttocks as you apply palm pressure to the opposite thigh.

   After holding this position for 5 to 10 seconds, slowly release the stretch, bringing your partner's feet back down to the floor. Then do the same stretch on the other leg for balance.

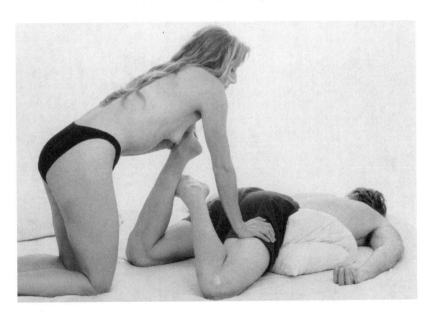

3. **Leg on Lap Shiatsu:** Lift your partner's leg up from the ankle, sliding the side of your knee underneath your partner's thigh. Use your elbow and forearm to massage your partner's lower back. Lean into the body, but be careful to stay off the spine.

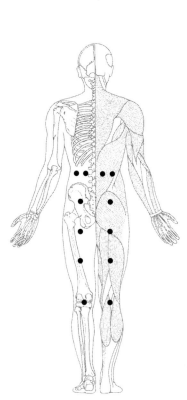

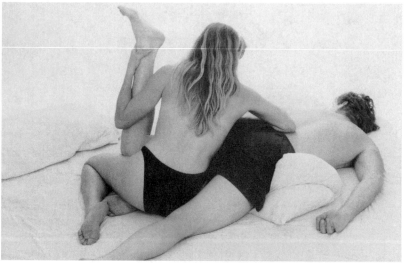

Roll your forearm up and down the back and the buttocks. Roll both your forearms on the thigh in front of you. Then turn around to work on your partner's other leg.

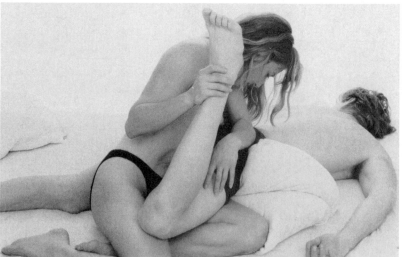

4. **The Chair:** This is a convenient way to work on the lower back. Bend your partner's legs to a 90-degree angle at the knees. With the bottoms of your partner's feet facing up, use them as a seat to sit on. Straddle your partner's thighs, placing your hands on the buttocks. Slowly squat down, placing your butt on the bottoms of your partner's feet.

As you balance your body's weight, use palm pressure on your partner's lower back. Walk your thumbs up and down on the large ropelike muscles that run parallel to the spine. Apply palm pressure to your partner's sacrum, the large flat bone at the base of the spine, above the crack of the buttocks. Finish this back massage by lightly gliding your fingertips up and down all areas of the buttocks, back, shoulders, head, arms, and hands, tantalizing your partner with sensual pleasure.

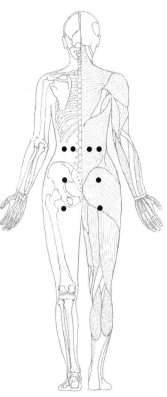

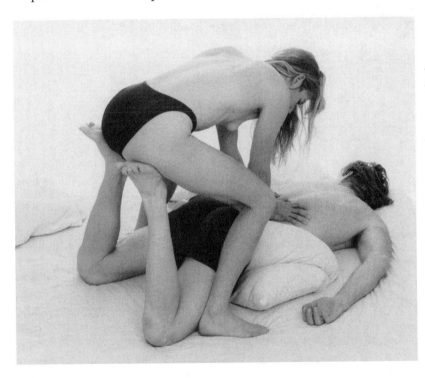

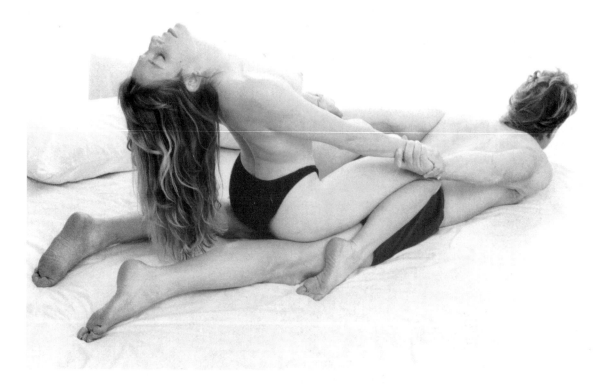

5. **Body Bowed Ski Ride:** Straddling your partner's hips, squat down, gently placing your knees on your partner's buttocks muscles. Make sure your knees do not contact any bony structures.

Place your toes on the floor beside your partner's knees. With your partner's hands by his or her sides, ask your partner to grasp your wrists as you slowly kneel on the buttocks. Ask your partner to bring his or her head all the way back as you both inhale, leaning backward into a dynamic stretch with your arms fully extended. Take two or three long deep breaths together in this position. Then slowly lower your partner with his or her head resting on its side. Tell your partner to relax completely.

Caution: If you have a weak back or a serious medical problem or injury, consult with your doctor before trying this powerful exercise.

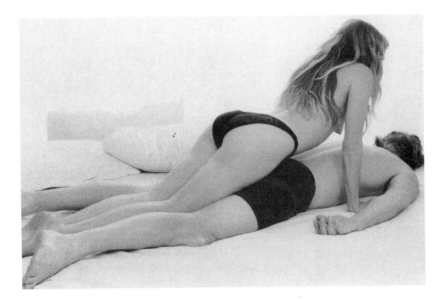

6. **Collapsing on Top of Your Lover:** Last, bring your knees between your partner's thighs and slowly lie down, fitting your partner's buttocks into your belly. Then place the side of your head against your partner's body. Bend your arms, comfortably placing your hands on your partner's shoulders, kneading the muscles slowly and gently. Take long, deep breaths into your heart as you let yourself completely relax.

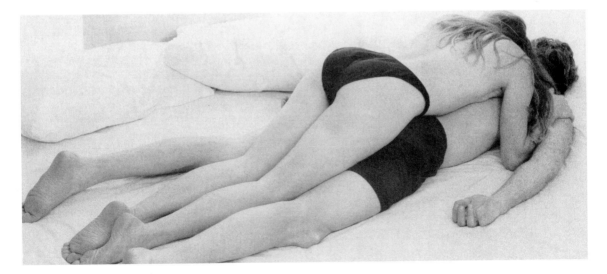

Chapter 12

ACUPRESSURE FOR THE AFTERGLOW

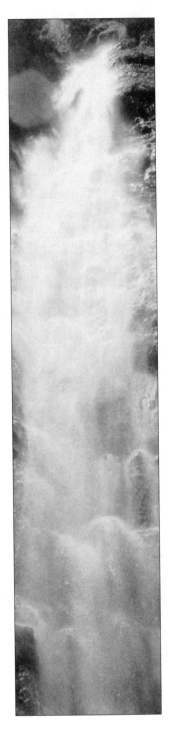

O rgasms create a dynamic interplay within the body's muscles, nerves, blood flow, and hormones. During orgasm, intense muscular contractions occur in the pelvic region. The body's own painkillers, the neurochemical substances known as endorphins, become more active in the nervous system. Increased circulation quickly distributes these natural body chemicals. The stimulation of orgasm affects the brain and even affects mood and consciousness.

In the Asian worldview, orgasms also cause the kidneys to release tremendous amounts of vital energy, or chi. The practices in this chapter are designed to heighten your experiences after orgasm, to enhance, transmute, and heighten this energy flow, to enable your sexual juices to be a healing force in your life, and to contribute to your spiritual growth. By holding points on each other, you create an outlet for the healing energy to circulate throughout your bodies.

Maximize Physical Contact

Making contact from head to toe immediately after orgasm greatly increases the flow of healing energy throughout your bodies. Embracing each other with maximum contact connects all the vital energy centers, or chakras. Each chakra governs major nerve plexuses, functioning as a transmitter for bioelectrical energy. When you and your partner's pelvic bones, bellies, and breastbones are aligned, your chakras are touching. Place your feet on your partner's feet, and bring your temples together as well.

Embrace in Stillness

After orgasm, it is rewarding to be still and quiet together, simply embracing each other and experiencing fully the release of energy. Consider meditating with your partner in a full-body embrace after you both have had orgasms. A couple's meditation requires your bodies to be still, calm, quiet, and serene. Human energy flows most strongly when the spine is stationary.

Breathe Deeply in Sync

Deep breathing supplements your energy and enhances its flow. When a couple breathes deeply together, they calm, balance, and harmonize each other. Conscious deep breathing not only attunes them to increased sensual pleasures but also transmits inner spiritual experiences. Thus, arousing sexual energy can provide a transcendental jump-start. When you train yourself to breathe slowly and deeply into your erotic feelings, you ignite your sexual energy by oxygenating your blood and body tissues. If you continue to breathe long, slow, deep breaths together after an orgasm, the climax will be intensified, and you will experience a profound feeling of oneness.

Deeply Relax

Your consciousness changes when you relax together. After an orgasm, you may experience waves of relaxation. Freed from struggling against muscular tensions, your mind is able to go off into an expansive realm yet remain fully aware of the present moment. This state of mind has refreshing, healing effects that revitalize the body's physical and mental capabilities.

Use Acupressure

A full embrace naturally contacts many acupressure points. Since these points are the gateways for healing energy, consciously holding them on each other after making love amplifies the power of the flow.

PLEASURE POINTS

After orgasm, you can hold any combination of acupressure points on yourself or on your partner. Since each orgasm produces a unique transcendent experience, you may hold a different combination of points each time your partner has an orgasm, creating a wide range of ecstatic spiritual experiences. Although you can hold any acupressure points safely on your partner during and after orgasm, the following combinations are particularly powerful.

Long Strength (GV 1) and
One Hundred Meeting (GV 20)

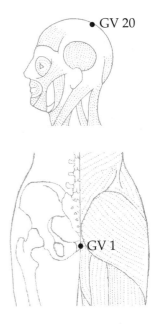

Location: Long Strength (GV 1) is located in a slight indentation at the base of the tailbone. One Hundred Meeting (GV 20) is located in the hollow of the skull at the top of the back of the head. On infants, this point is often referred to as the soft spot.

Benefits: Holding these points on each other for at least 2 minutes after one or both of you has had an orgasm can create a heavenly feeling. When the top and bottom of the spinal cord are held simultaneously, cerebral spinal fluid circulates through the spine, conducting energy throughout the central nervous system. It also increases the flow of the life force through the meridians, sending healing energy through the entire body.

Directions: Place your middle finger in the upper crack of the buttocks on GV 1, under the tip of the tailbone. Gradually press into a small hollow in the bone. The GV 1 point is often quite sensitive when you make contact. Use your other hand on GV 20, in the indentation of the skull on the back top of the head.

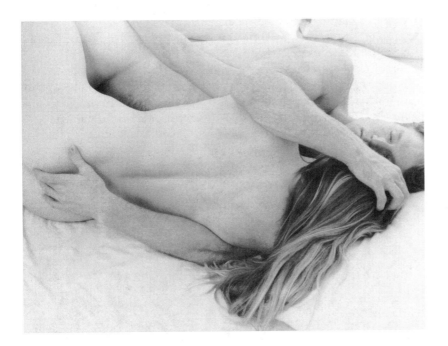

235

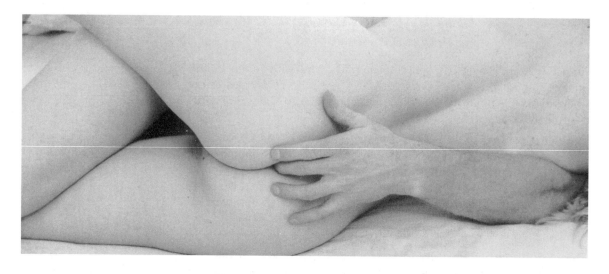

GV 20

GV 1

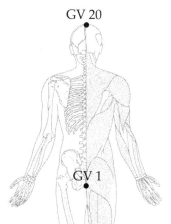

As you hold these points, make your embrace comfortable and cozy. Breathe slowly and deeply with your partner, keeping your bodies relaxed and still as you hold these points for several minutes.

As you breathe in deeply together with your eyes closed, imagine life energy coming into your heart. As you slowly exhale, imagine the energy in your body moving out through your arms, hands, and fingertips into your partner's vital nervous system.

Breathe deeply together. Focus on breathing in simultaneously, holding the breath for a few seconds, and exhaling slowly together as you hold each other's points lightly. Try to breathe this way for 3 to 5 minutes. Work your way up to 10 minutes or more to gain the full spiritual impact of this powerful couple's meditation.

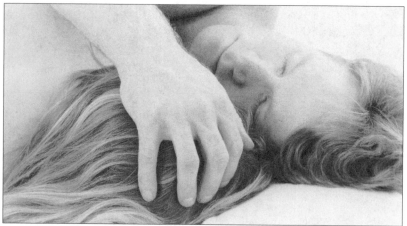

Sea of Vitality (B 23 and B 47) *with Heavenly Pillar* (B 10) *and/or*
Gates of Consciousness (GB 20)

Benefits: B 23 and B 47 fortify the reproductive system and adrenal glands. These are especially vital points to hold after an orgasm since they replenish the kidneys—where sexual energy is stored.

Directions: While lying on top of, beneath, or beside your partner, one hand can hold both sides of the lower back at once. Cup your hand, placing your fingertips on one side, while the heel of your hand presses the other side of the lower back.

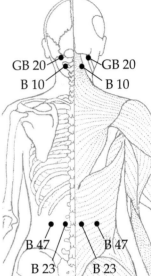

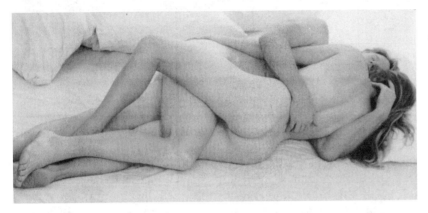

Place your other hand on the back of your partner's neck to press B 10 and/or GB 20. Steadily squeeze the ropelike muscles of your partner's neck, using your fingertips on one side of the neck and the heel of your hand on the other to press B 10. You can also press GB 20 underneath the base of your partner's skull.

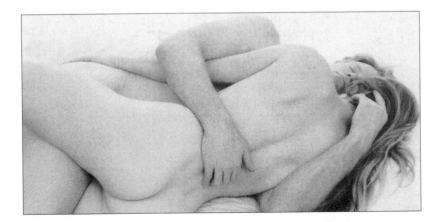

237

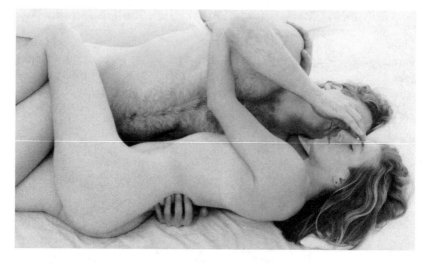

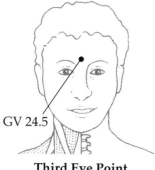

GV 24.5

Third Eye Point

As you hold these points, breathe deeply in sync with your partner for a few minutes. Then gradually take one hand off of either the neck or lower back. To give your partner an extra uplifting feeling, place the free hand lightly on the Third Eye point between the eyebrows, using the pad of your middle finger. Keeping your fingertip still, maintain a constant contact with the Third Eye point. Holding this point is excellent for releasing mental stress and activating the pituitary, the master endocrine gland. Holding the neck or lower back supports the major curves of the spine and relaxes the nervous system. Lightly touching the Third Eye point often results in a transformative healing experience.

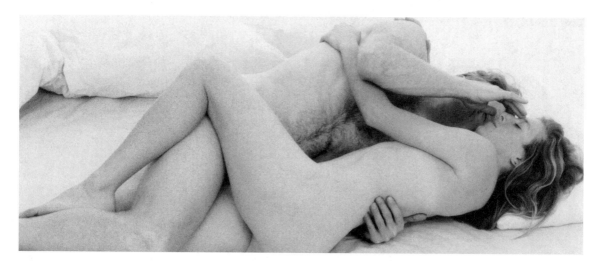

Inner Gates (P 6) *and Labor Palace* (P 8)

These acupressure points are especially nurturing, soothing, and rejuvenating for your sexual relationship. Holding them after an orgasm reestablishes your emotional balance and strongly connects your romantic and erotic selves, harmonizing your heart and mind.

Whether you are on the top or the bottom after your partner comes, grasp hold of P 6 on both sides, 3 finger-widths from the wrist crease on the center of the inside of the forearm. As you press this point firmly with your thumb, place your fingertips directly behind. Hold for a minute or two as you breathe slowly and deeply.

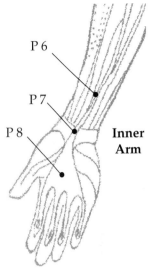

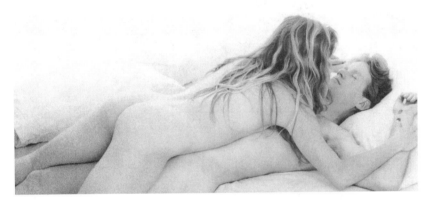

Reposition your thumbs to P 8, in the center of your partner's palm. With your feet, make contact with both of your partner's feet as you focus again on taking long, slow, deep breaths.

With the palms of your hands touching, interlace your fingers together. Bring your feet in contact with both of your partner's feet. With your eyes closed, synchronize your breath, taking long, slow, deep breaths together. Feel your bodies merge into an experience of oneness—the unified feeling essential for spiritual growth.

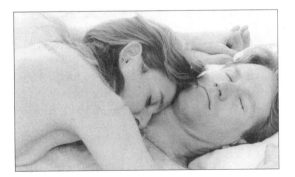

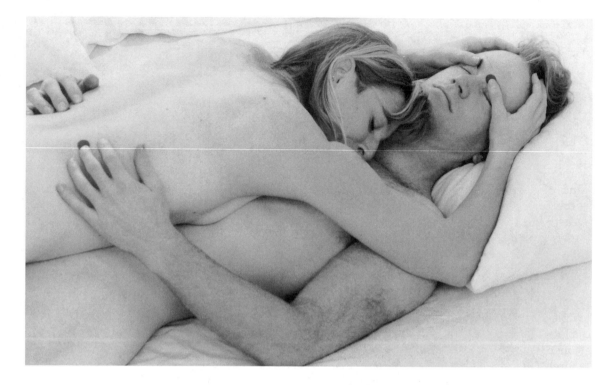

Sea of Vitality (B 23 and B 47) *and Drilling Bamboo* (B 2)

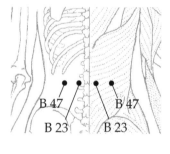

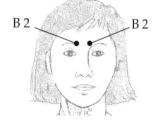

Support your partner's lower back, holding B 23 and B 47 to benefit the reproductive system and adrenal glands. While lying beside your partner, one hand can hold both sides of the lower back and press both of these points at once. Cup your hand, placing your fingers on one side and the heel of your hand on the other side of the lower back, and squeeze gently.

With your thumb and middle finger of your other hand on the upper inside ridge of your partner's eye socket, press B 2. Gently and steadily press upward into the slight indentations of the eye socket. To give your partner an extra uplifting feeling, let your index finger lightly touch the Third Eye point, between the eyebrows.

Holding these points on the forehead releases mental stress and activates the pituitary gland. Holding the lower back supports the body's vital energy system. Using this mind/body point combination along with long, deep breathing often results in a transformative experience.

Third Eye (GV 24.5), One Hundred Meeting (GV 20), Sea of Tranquility (CV 17), and Sea of Vitality (CV 6)

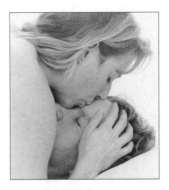

During or soon after your partner's orgasm, passionately kiss the center of the forehead between the eyebrows. Gradually create a firm, steady suction with your lips for 1 or 2 minutes as you continue to breathe deeply.

Lie on your side, snuggling close to your partner. Use the hand closer to the ground to reach up, lightly touching GV 20 in the center of the top of your partner's head. Place the fingertips of your free hand at CV 17, on the center of your partner's breastbone at the level of the heart. Fit your fingertips into the indentations of the skull and breastbone. Breathe slow, quiet, long, deep breaths while holding these two points for a couple of minutes.

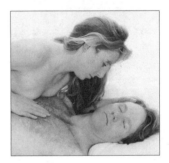

As you hold the top of your partner's head (GV 20) lightly, your other hand moves from the breastbone down to the center of your partner's lower abdominal area, 3 finger-widths directly below the navel (CV 6). Hold this point firmly with the palm of your hand for a couple of minutes as you both breathe deeply into your lower bellies.

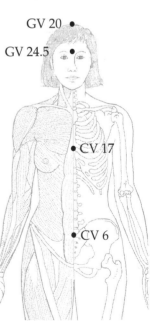

Holding these acupressure points after orgasm raises the consciousness of both lovers. Cuddle and embrace, wrapping your arms securely around each other, making firm contact with both of your partner's feet. Breathe slowly and deeply in sync, merging your bodies into one pulsating vibrant being.

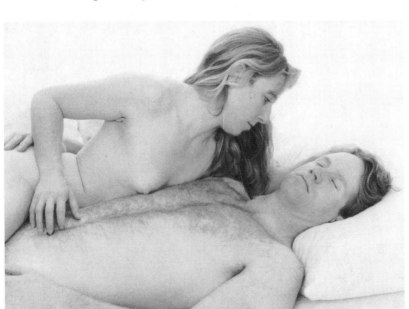

GV 20

GV 24.5

CV 17

CV 6

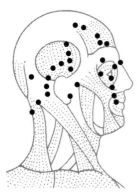

COMBINING POINTS AND POSITIONS

Once you and your partner become comfortable holding these points after orgasm, you will find that each point combination creates a unique transcendent experience, both ecstatic and spiritual in nature.

The following six combinations are particularly powerful. Hold at least two points at once from the following sets:

- **Head and facial points:** B 1–B 9, St 1–St 6, GV 25–GV 27, CV 24
- **Neck and skull points:** GV 15–GV 24.5, GB 1–GB 20, B 10
- **Breastbone points:** CV 17–CV 19
- **Lower abdominal points:** CV 2–CV 6

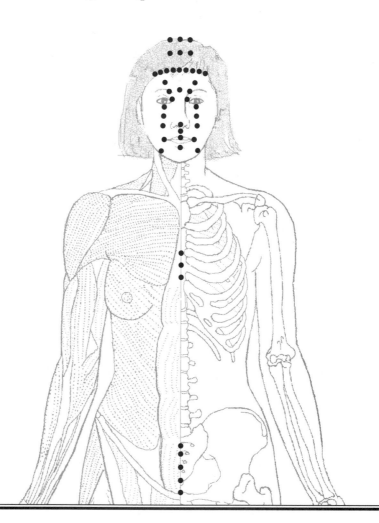

FOR THE AFTERGLOW

- **Back points**

   Lower back: B 23, B 47, GV 3–GV 5

   Sacral points: B 27–B 34

   Tailbone: GV 1

   Upper back: B 13–B 17, B 37–B 41

- **Feet/ankle points:** K 1–K 8, Sp 1–Sp 6, Lv 1–Lv 5

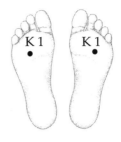

Passionate embraces stimulate these potent back points.

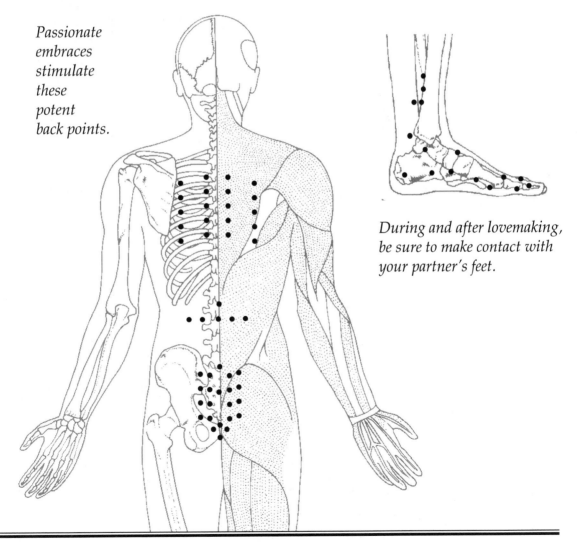

During and after lovemaking, be sure to make contact with your partner's feet.

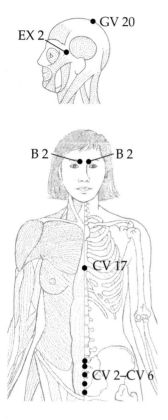

POINTS TO HOLD WHILE SPOONING

When you are spooning your partner, with your front facing your partner's back, try holding these acupressure points.

- **Head-Heart Combination:** Hold GV 20 on the back top of your partner's head, along with CV 17 in the center of the breastbone. These points are in slight indentations of the bone structure.

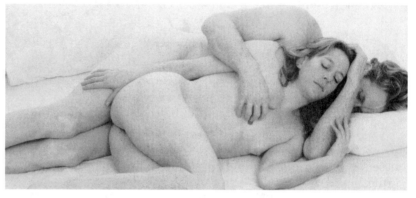

- **Temple and Lower Belly Combination:** Raise the arm underneath you up beside your head with the elbow bent to hold your partner's temple point (Ex 2) in the indentation outside of the eyebrow. Place the palm of your other hand firmly on your partner's lower abdominal points (CV 2–CV 6), between the belly button and pubic bone. Breathe deeply with your partner as you hold these points with your eyes closed for several minutes.

Note: The person being spooned in front can place his or her hands over his or her partner's hands to reinforce the contact.

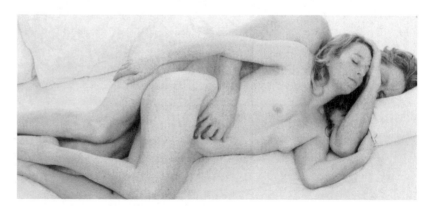

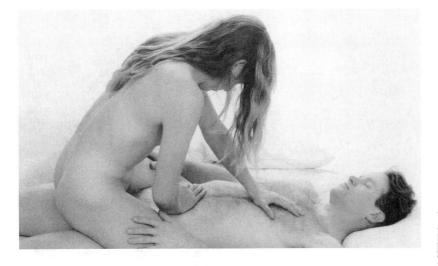

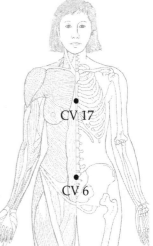

Straddling the Pelvis

These combinations can be comfortable to hold while straddling your partner in a kneeling position.

- **Heart-Belly Combination:** Place the palms of your hands on the center of the breastbone to press CV 17 and on the center of your partner's lower belly to hold CV 6.

- **Wrists:** Use a moderate amount of pressure to press P 7 and P 8, on the inside of your partner's wrist, and in the center of the palm of the hand.

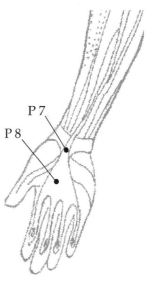

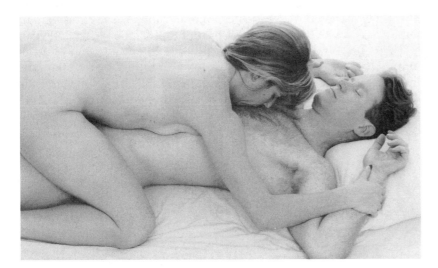

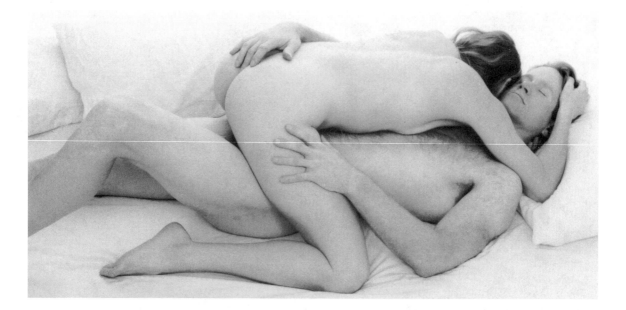

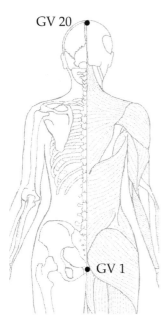

GV 20

GV 1

- **Top of the Head with the Tailbone:** As you lie on top of your partner in a kneeling position, bring one hand up to the top of your partner's head to hold the One Hundred Meeting point (GV 20). Use your other hand to press the base of your partner's tailbone, Long Strength (GV 1). Remain still, and keep your eyes closed while you breathe deeply with your partner for several minutes to discover the benefits.

During an orgasm, your verbal expression of love can be unconditionally accepted. Affectionate communication during this ecstatic time goes directly to the heart instead of to the rational, analytic part of the brain. When you tell your partner of her beauty and radiance during her orgasm, the affirming words of your love expand her state of ecstasy. When you tell your male partner how much you value and love him during his orgasm, the words bypass the judgments of his mind and go straight to his heart. Thus, the ecstasy of orgasm opens the heart for reaching your partner's innermost being.

Chapter 13

TROUBLESHOOTING:
ACUPRESSURE FOR SEXUAL PROBLEMS

*S*everal years ago I worked with Shelly and Bob, a couple who had a long history of sexual problems. Bob had been through extended periods of high stress as he tried to build up the company he had started. Reaching his business goals required long work hours and diverted him from spending quality time with his wife. This triggered within Shelly what she identified as "abandonment issues," which she connected to events in her childhood. (For example, her alcoholic father had been unreliable or absent when she needed him.)

After the first year or so of marriage, their sex life dwindled. Bob began to suffer from premature ejaculation, while Shelly's desire for sex became inhibited, no doubt partly in response to her frustration with Bob's lack of involvement in their relationship.

I worked with Shelly and Bob for about a year. After talking with them about their problems, I did acupressure on them and showed them how to do acupressure on each other. I taught them several couple's exercises and self-help techniques. They learned to give each other satisfying full-body treatments for deeply relaxing with each other. The more I worked with them, the more they seemed to enjoy the acupressure sessions. Bob even surprised Shelly by coming home early from work in anticipation of their acupressure. Their sessions left them feeling loving and playful—and they were able to enjoy being together in a way they had not experienced in years. Eventually, their sexual problems were alleviated.

Admittedly, the results did not come quickly and easily. There were setbacks related to emotional and even practical considerations—Bob needed to overcome a tendency to press too quickly and forcefully on the points, while Shelly needed to learn how to lean her weight into points when applying acupressure to Bob. The couple complemented their acupressure practices with weekly visits to a

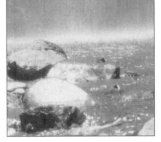

We have to acknowledge all the old beliefs, judgments, and attitudes that have kept us from experiencing our true sexuality.

—Shakti Gawain
Living in the Light

psychotherapist, who helped them work on the underlying personal issues in their relationship. In the final analysis, however, both Bob and Shelly felt that acupressure was an important component in reestablishing a satisfying sexual life.

Inhibited sexual desire and premature ejaculation are two of the most common sexual problems couples face today. These and other common sexual problems, such as difficulty achieving erection or orgasm, may all be helped by certain acupressure techniques.

Walk into your terror

to learn its nature. It

will be less painful if

you do not turn away.

Stay with the feeling

itself, with no attempt

to give it structure. It is

structure that causes

terror, not experience.

You will see.

—Emmanuel
(Pat Rodegast)

INHIBITED SEXUAL DESIRE

Inhibited sexual desire is simply the inability to enjoy normal sexual activities. It affects both men and women. Until recently, the condition was popularly known as "frigidity," which is now recognized as an inappropriate term. As the American Medical Association notes in its *Encyclopedia of Medicine*, "The term has been used almost exclusively with reference to women and is now being discouraged because of its negative connotations—blaming a woman for something that may exist only in the mind of her partner." The *Encyclopedia* also distinguishes between inhibited sexual desire and anorgasmia—failure to achieve orgasm.

Inhibited sexual desire is often the result of sexual wounds. Once any part of your body is wounded, it becomes vulnerable and hypersensitive, needing extreme protection. During the initial state of shock, the muscles, tendons, and ligaments surrounding the area tense up as a protective response. Often this constriction remains long after the physical wound heals. The scars can hamper the body for years. Therapeutic massage and bodywork, along with counseling or therapy, can release the chronic tension.

When a man or woman is sexually wounded, the trauma may affect both body and mind. This is because there is a strong connection between the genitals and emotions, a link acknowledged in traditional Chinese medicine for thousands of years. (Practitioners of traditional Chinese medicine note that the kidney, pericardium, and triple warmer energy pathways connect the emotions to sexuality. The pericardium is often referred to as the protector of the heart, linking emotions to the genitals.)

A person's body can become sexually unresponsive due to past wounds from childhood sexual abuse, incest, rape, forceful male fingering and entry, premature intercourse, saying yes when no is meant, guilty masturbation, abortion, cesarean section, or hysterectomy.

Social pressures can hit women especially hard. A woman may feel driven to fake an orgasm to please her mate's ego. Fearing that her partner will feel responsible for her nonorgasmic condition, she may settle for an inauthentic sexual relationship rather than upset him or risk losing him. She may also not want to appear aggressive or selfish in asking for what feels good.

Of course, inhibited sexual desire may also result from physical problems. Painful intercourse may have a medical cause, such as pelvic endometriosis or ligamental tears that occurred during childbirth, so it is important for a woman who experiences it to be examined by a doctor.

To determine whether their inhibited sexual desire has an organic cause, men and women should begin by asking themselves the following questions:

- Are you able to bring yourself to orgasm?
- Are you more likely to have an orgasm on vacation?
- Are there certain partners, environments, or circumstances that cause you to experience orgasm without effort?

If you answered yes to any of these questions, you probably do not have a physical problem. Your sexual discomfort may be due to stress or an emotional cause, which can be healed over time through a combination of supportive, somatic psychotherapy and regular private acupressure sessions.

Sexual unresponsiveness may be the body's wisdom speaking. When a person feels deeply supported, safe, and able to trust another human being, the body often rediscovers its sexual responsiveness.

Even if you have a loving partner, self-healing is the most important element in overcoming inhibited sexual desire. Focus on the following:

Take Responsibility for Your Body

Learn the basics about your sexual responses and the techniques for deriving sexual satisfaction.

Explore the Acupressure Points

Use acupressure on the points that benefit the sexual-reproductive system. These points are presented in Chapters 6 and 7. Also practice the daily stretches in Chapter 3, increasing your self-awareness and healing.

Socio-cultural influence more often than not places a woman in a position in which she must adapt, sublimate, inhibit, or even distort her natural capacity to function sexually in order to fulfill her genetically assigned role. Herein lies the source of women's sexual dysfunction.

—William Masters
and Virginia Johnson
Human Sexual Inadequacy

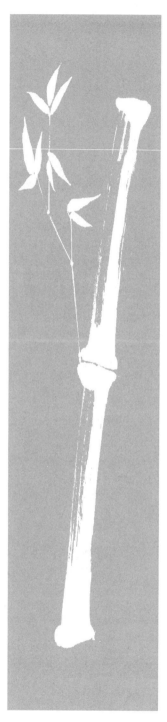

Celebrate Your Body

Let go of your "nonsexual" image of yourself. We are all sexual; it is part of being alive. Spend time bathing, touching, being touched, and enjoying your sexuality.

Give Pleasure to Your Body

"When you can do kindly things to yourself then you know what it is to be able to love yourself," notes Gary Zukav in *Seat of the Soul*. Sex therapists recommend that people with inhibited sexual desire achieve sexual pleasure through self-stimulation before engaging with a partner. If the person has tremendous guilt about masturbation, this work can be especially difficult.

Feel Good About Your Body

Self-consciousness can lead to obsessive criticism of your own sexual performance. You may be self-conscious about sounds, intimate expressions, and even body movements. It is crucial to let go of such self-consciousness, of irrational obsessions and harsh judgments about your body (about thinness, for example). The exercises and stretches throughout this book will enable you to feel better about your body and thus decrease your self-consciousness.

Discover Your Sexual Preferences

Pleasure yourself in order to learn what is sexually arousing to you. Get to know your genitals. Experiment with a variety of touches (light stroking, teasing, gentle rubbing, firm rubbing) until you know what pleases your body most.

Cultivate an Appreciation for Your Partner

Acknowledge the value of your relationship. Take a moment to express gratitude for the qualities, actions, and attitudes that you appreciate about your partner. Acknowledge the qualities and habits of your partner that attract you to him or her.

Practice Acupressure Massage

The acupressure routines in this book refocus attention on intimacy. No longer is orgasm the main goal. As a result of taking more time to be intimate, couples:

- create more special time for playing and enjoying each other's bodies
- have longer periods of arousal
- feel each pleasurable sensation at its maximum intensity
- enjoy long-term pleasurable sensations throughout the body
- respond to their body signals and immediate experiences rather than remotely evaluating performance

Experiment with Taking Charge Yourself

Actively pursue your own sexual satisfaction. Use your partner's body to bring you pleasure. Do only what feels good to you. Become an active participant. Each partner must feel free to express wishes, desires, and needs in his or her unique way, as they occur, spontaneously and naturally, rather than rely on gender stereotypes or some "authoritative" sex guide.

Tell Your Partner What Works for You

Tell him or her what is pleasurable and what is painful. Your partner won't know what you need if you don't communicate. Teach your partner the details of how to stimulate you. Direct stimulation of the clitoris, for example, may be irritating or painful to some women. No one should tolerate pain or discomfort during sex.

Use a minimum of words. Simply show what you like. Place your hand over your partner's to signal more touch, less touch, or touch in another place. The pressure, direction, and rapidity are directed by you because it is your body. There is no shame in knowing your body intimately, then sharing it, exploring it, and guiding your partner in pleasuring it.

Lose Yourself in the Pleasure as it Rises Within Your Own Body

Focus on your own sexual pleasure. Let go of taking care of your partner. Feel what is happening in you instead of simply accommodating your partner's pattern. Lose yourself in the pleasure growing between you and your partner. For an acupressure routine to help to restore your body's sexual responsiveness, see Chapter 14.

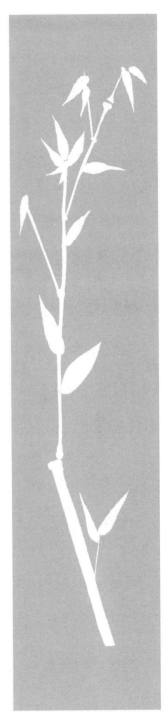

TOWARD SEXUAL HEALING

Acupressure's healing program for sexual problems involves three essential components. First, adopt a healthy lifestyle, including a balanced whole-foods diet, stress reduction, and daily exercise. Second, let go of old attitudes and expectations, all of your destructive patterns and baggage. These first two components are your sole responsibility; the third component involves collaboration with your partner.

Practice couple's exercises and full-body acupressure massages that refocus your attention on pleasurable sensations throughout your body. Eventually this will lead to a transformed experience of your sexuality. The stretches, exercises, and massage routines offered in this book refocus your attention naturally by touching all parts of your partner's body. No longer is each other's orgasm the central focus of making love.

POTENT POINTS FOR A BALANCED SEX LIFE

Chronic muscular tension in the abdominal and pelvic regions can contribute to sexual problems. When the pelvic muscles are chronically tense, circulation to the genitals decreases. Restrictive clothing, poor posture, lack of exercise, shoulder tension, and emotional upset may contribute to pelvic and abdominal tension. For potency, fertility, and sexual sensations to be as full and pleasurable as possible, the pelvic area must be flexible.

Pressing the acupressure points in the pelvic and abdominal areas increases the flow of blood and sensory impulses through the sexual-reproductive organs. Holding acupressure points on the kidney, liver, and spleen meridians also benefits the reproductive system. By increasing circulation and building overall health, acupressure fortifies your body's sexual functions. The points in the lower back and the base of the spine (the sacrum), for example, relieve imbalances in the uterus and prostate gland. The following acupressure points strengthen both the male and female sexual-reproductive systems.

It can be as important and necessary for a woman to enjoy sex as it is for her to enjoy her work, children, environment, food or recreational activities. It's just another potentially satisfying aspect of life.

—Lonnie G. Barbach
For Yourself

Sea of Vitality (B 23 and B 47)

Caution: Do not press on disintegrating discs or fractured or broken bones. If you have a weak back, a few minutes of stationary light touching instead of pressure can be very healing. See your doctor first if you have any questions or need medical advice.

Location: On the lower back (between the second and third lumbar vertebrae), two and four finger-widths away from the spine at waist level, in line with the belly button.

Benefits: Pressing these points relieves lower back aches, fatigue, reproductive problems, impotence, and premature ejaculation.

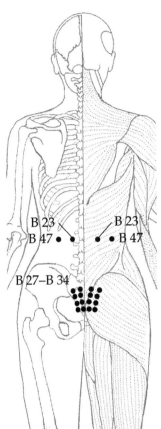

Sacral Points (B 27–B 34)

The points at the base of the spine also help relieve menstrual cramps and lower back pain. Steady, firm pressure on these sacral points—which are directly related to the reproductive system—can help impotence.

Point	Health Benefits
B 27, B 28	Relieves hip pain (especially in the sacroiliac joint), reproductive problems, and retention of urine
B 29, B 30	Relieves impotence, lumbago, sacral pain, and sciatica
B 31, B 32	Relieves lumbago and impotence
B 33, B 34	Relieves sterility, irregular vaginal discharge, and genital pain

Bubbling Spring (K 1)

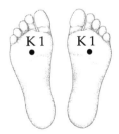

Location: On the center of the sole of the foot, at the base of the ball of the foot, between the two pads.

Benefits: Pressing this points relieves hot flashes as well as impotence.

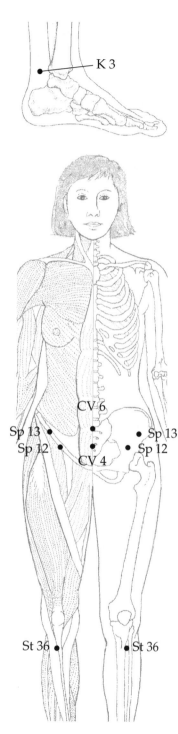

Bigger Stream (K 3)

Caution: This point should not be stimulated strongly after the third month of pregnancy.

Location: Midway between the inside anklebone and the Achilles tendon, in the back of the ankle.

Benefits: Holding this point relieves sexual tensions, semen leakage, and menstrual irregularity.

Sea of Energy (CV 6)

Location: Three finger-widths directly below the belly button.

Benefits: Holding this point relieves uro-reproductive problems, irregular vaginal discharge, irregular periods, and impotence; also strengthens the sexual-reproductive system.

Gate of Origin (CV 4)

Location: Four finger-widths directly below the belly button.

Benefits: Holding this point relieves impotence, uro-reproductive problems, irregular vaginal discharge, irregular menstrual periods, and urinary incontinence.

Rushing Door (Sp 12) *and* Mansion Cottage (Sp 13)

Location: In the pelvic area, in the middle of the crease where the leg joins the trunk of the body.

Benefits: Holding these points is particularly good for relieving groin pain, impotence, and menstrual cramps.

Three Mile Point (St 36)

Location: Four finger-widths below the kneecap, one finger-width on the outside of the shinbone. If you are on the correct spot, a muscle will flex as you move your foot up and down.

Benefits: Holding this point strengthens the whole body, especially the muscles, and aids the sexual-reproductive system.

You do not have to use all of these points. Using just one or two of them whenever you have a free hand can be effective.

Difficulty Getting an Erection

According to William Masters and Virginia Johnson, your sexual functioning is a result of the interaction between the physical health of your reproductive system and your values and attitudes toward sex. The two most common male sexual problems are difficulty getting an erection (impotence) and premature ejaculation. If you suffer from difficulty getting an erection, first consult your doctor to see if you have an underlying organic or physical condition. Contributing causes of impotence include excessive use of alcohol or drugs, diabetes, and nerve damage. Impotence is frequently a side effect of some medications. If your doctor finds no physical dysfunction, therapy and education about sex to correct misinformation and dispel fear often make a difference.

Each individual has his or her own level of sexual need, of balance of sexual activity. Like any activity, sex can be overdone. An excess of sexual activity can dissipate or drain a man's reserve energies, resulting in temporary impotence.

Essential Dietary Considerations

Most men go through periods of time when their penis doesn't respond due to stress factors, the consumption of sugar or alcohol, preoccupations, worries, and other causes. Even when a man wants to make love, his penis can have a mind of its own. At these times, soft entry techniques can be useful. After thoroughly arousing his partner, the man makes a snug ring around the base of his penis with his thumb and index fingers. After a few minutes this firm hold will stiffen his penis, enabling more blood to accumulate into it. During this time he breathes slowly and deeply through his nose (if possible) as he slowly directs and manipulates his soft penis into his partner's vagina. With patience and persistence, his soft penis will not only find its way inside but will become hard in response to his partner's excitement. The soft entry method can be surprisingly satisfying and rewarding for both sexes.

The penis is an amazingly sensitive sexual organ, affected by what you think and worry about, as well as what you are attracted to. It is also affected by what you eat. Among the most common dietary considerations, according to many alternative health practitioners, are the following:

At one time or another, most men suffer from temporary impotence. That is probably putting it too strongly. What we mean is that at one time or another most men think that they want to make love only to find that the body is not willing.

—Jolan Chang
The Tao of Love and Sex

255

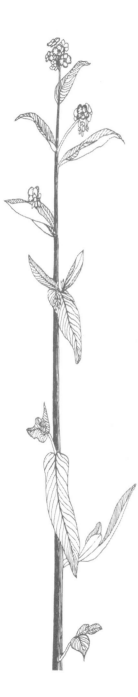

Avoid Eating Foods Containing Excessive Sugar

One of the most common causes of impotence is from overeating candy bars, sodas, frostings, ice cream, and chocolates. Try to stay away from these foods—they weaken your reproductive system.

Sugar is a major enemy of the kidneys as well as a potential cause of impotence and premature ejaculation. Metabolizing sugar significantly strains and taxes the adrenal glands, located directly on top of the kidneys.

Avoid Alcoholic Drinks

Some men's sexual responsiveness is weakened by drinking alcohol; some is not. Experiment to see if alcohol affects yours.

Imbibing excess fluids—especially alcohol—taxes the kidneys, requiring them to work harder. Contrary to Western thinking, drinking too much water every day is detrimental to the kidneys. For proper balance, drink when you are thirsty, taking in small amounts of liquid throughout the day. The common belief that you "cleanse" the body by "flushing" it with large amounts of fluids can contribute to impotence.

Eat More Fish

Fish contains a high concentration of minerals and vitamins that can strengthen the male sexual-reproductive system. Oysters in particular are a rich source of zinc, which is possibly a key mineral for strengthening many sexual functions.

Impotence and Emotional Stress

Emotions such as fear, insecurity, and performance anxiety can diminish a man's sexual vitality. In some relationships, impotence is due to a lack of mutual responsiveness. Tension and anxiety can result from an absence of openness and communication. Emotional work encourages openness, trust, communication, and the letting go of expectations and judgments—all of which can greatly improve sexual relations.

Men who are angry but repress it are more likely to become impotent or to ejaculate prematurely. Repressed anger is common in our culture, which advocates strict morals but rarely observes them. Repressed anger affects the liver by blocking the liver meridian, which travels through the scrotum, thus impeding a man's ability to be aroused.

Dependency and fear are related to the kidney meridian, a pathway directly connected to the sexual-reproductive system and therefore to potency. Impotence can be related to feelings of guilt and self-doubt. Fear and insecurity as well as the other extreme—egocentricity and a foolhardy attempt to show fearlessness—can all cause interpersonal problems, weaken the kidneys, and affect potency.

Organic Causes of Impotence

Cold

The kidneys are temperature-sensitive. The kidneys and the sexual-reproductive system can be damaged by prolonged exposure to extreme cold. Lack of warm clothing or bedding during cold weather, especially over a period of time, can cause this type of organic impotence. Similarly, eating cold foods, such as cold drinks or ice cream, especially in cold weather, can damage the kidneys' energy reserves.

In moderation, however, cold can strengthen the body as a whole, the kidneys' energy reserves, and the sexual organs. Taking a cold shower for a few minutes each day can build kidney energy.

Fatigue and Chronic Stress

Traditionally, winter is a time to retreat and reserve your energy. If you are excessively outgoing during the winter months, overconsume sweets, and foolishly expend your energy reserves, you may damage your vital energy systems, resulting in chronic fatigue, lower back problems, or any other illness. Nurture your energy as you would plants in a garden: cultivate in the spring; develop and strengthen in the summer; gather and store in the fall; and conserve during the winter. Living in harmony with the seasons and the elements of nature is important for maintaining health and essential for developing potency.

Lower Back Problems

Since the kidneys are located in the lower back, a stiff or weak lower back can affect them. Many people have lower back problems, and they may also have kidney problems or sexual or reproductive difficulties. It's important to use acupressure points and gentle stretches in this area.

Medications

Many prescription and over-the-counter drugs may adversely affect sexual functioning.

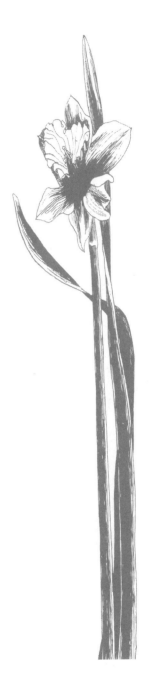

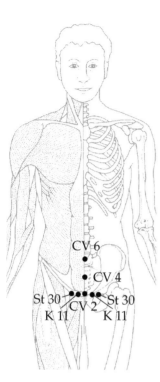

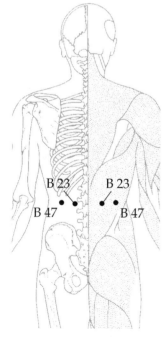

How to Promote an Erection

The following exercises and self-acupressure techniques are most effective when practiced on a regular basis in conjunction with diet and lifestyle improvements. If you have difficulty getting an erection, practice them three times a day.

Vigorously Rub Your Pubic Bone

This will stimulate three important acupressure points on the pubic bone that strengthen the male reproductive system: K 11, CV 2, and St 30. Simply make a fist, and briskly rub across your pubic bone for 1 minute. You can do this with your clothes on or off. Rub briskly enough that you create heat in order to stimulate these potent points.

Rub Your Lower Back Briskly

Using the backs of both of your hands, rub your lower back rapidly for 1 minute. This stimulates points in your lower back (B 23 and B 47) and fortifies your kidneys, where sexual energy is stored.

Perform the Lower Belly Press

Place your fingertips one inch above the center of your pubic bone. Apply firm pressure to CV 4 as you breathe deeply for 1 minute.

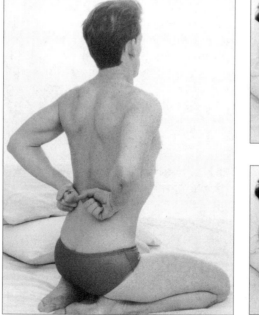

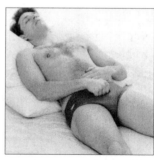

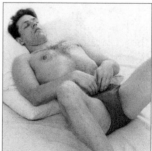

Stretch Your Inner Thigh Muscles

Stand with your legs spread wide apart. Slowly bend over, touching your hands to the floor in front of you. Bend one leg, bringing your weight over it to stretch your opposite leg's inner thigh. Then do the other side. Continue to stretch for 1 minute as you open up the meridians that travel into the genital region.

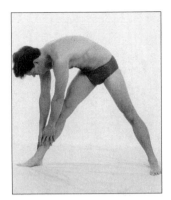

Practice the Acupressure Healing Program (See Chapter 14)

This is an excellent routine for someone who has difficulty getting an erection. Alternatively, you and your partner can practice this shorter, quicker version:

Lie on your back, feet flat on the floor and legs spread comfortably apart. Your partner kneels between your knees and places her hands on the insides of your thighs, on the Joy of Living point (Lv 9). Breathe deeply into your belly as she slowly glides her fingertips up the insides of your thighs through points Lv 10, Lv 11, and Lv 12. She places the head of your penis on your lower belly. Then she places the heels of her hands in your groin and presses the Rushing Door and Mansion Cottage points (Sp 12 and Sp 13), with her fingertips on top of your penis. She holds this for 1 minute as you continue to breathe deeply into your belly. Once the Rushing Door points are open, sexual energy can flow through the genitals. She lightly caresses the inner thighs through your scrotum up to the head of your penis. As she repeats this stroke several times, she may vary the pathway of her touch to enliven the entire area between your legs. Make pelvic movements and continue breathing deeply into your belly as she intensifies the speed of each caress.

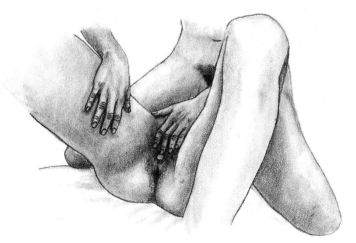

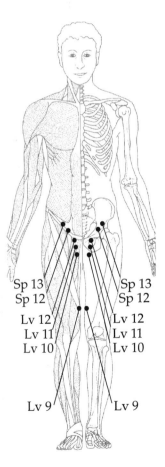

Premature Ejaculation

John, a salesman, came to me looking for help with a problem he had been trying to deal with for many years. When he had intercourse with his wife, he would either have difficulty getting an erection or he would ejaculate almost immediately without control. "The thing just doesn't work anymore. Is there anything you can do for me? Most of the time I don't let my wife touch me—it makes my body cringe." I showed him how to use several acupressure points along with some therapeutic exercises.

We worked together on weekly assigned exercises for five months. During the first two weeks, he seemed to have no results; his penis responded no differently to his wife. The more he experimented with the acupressure points, the love positions, and the exercises for intimacy (see Chapter 4), however, the more comfortable he got. He began to feel his body relax. His new way of being completely changed his outlook on his sexual relationship, enabled him to relax and nurture himself, and he gained much more intimacy with his wife.

Unfortunately, these changes didn't affect his actual sexual performance. He went through a lot of emotional pain and some depression about his problem. Finally, after practicing deep breathing exercises and spending time relaxing with his wife, John felt a shift in his sexual chemistry. He actually let his wife touch him again—and he enjoyed it.

"I thought it was my role to 'do it' to my wife," he said. "The pressures created within me, especially when I couldn't 'get it up,' made me so tense I couldn't handle her light caresses. It's strange how I'm able to relax and receive her touch now. Not having to be on top of her and in control (which didn't work to satisfy her anyway) opened up a whole new world for us."

To prevent premature ejaculation, stay relaxed and calm, slow down, giving everything time, slow and deepen your breathing, and let go of sexual expectations.

—Sun-Nu Ching
The Classic of the Plain Girl

Causes of Premature Ejaculation

Expectations and performance anxiety often cause physical tension. When a man's body is exhausted or weakened by stress, he may experience premature ejaculation. Acupressure releases this stress and tension, allowing the energy to flow freely, and it can restore sexual endurance.

The truth is that every man ejaculates prematurely from time to time, and all men at some point in their lives experience periods of premature ejaculation.

Premature ejaculation is not the same as impotence, though it may lead to erective failure. With premature ejaculation, erection happens, but the man ejaculates outside of his partner, or soon after entering her. He often feels inadequate, and his partner is often left unsatisfied.

Other contributing causes of premature ejaculation and impotence include cultural pressures and the partner's expectations. Men who ejaculate prematurely, without conscious control, may also unconsciously be gripped by worries or stress over which they have no control.

Successful intercourse is an important goal for most heterosexual couples. It often creates great expectations and anxiety around a sexual situation. Men in particular are taught a performance-based attitude about sex, and they often measure their sex life by how often they achieve the goal of "getting it on" or simply "getting off." This narrow focus places men in a precarious situation. When a man discovers that he has limited control over his erection, his anxiety soars. He may view his penis and sexuality as malfunctioning. Unfortunately, this lack of control and performance anxiety can escalate fears about intimacy and openness with women.

To deal with uncontrolled ejaculation, a man usually becomes fixated on "holding back" the ejaculation, to slow it down. This deliberate blocking of sexual stimuli can itself lead to erective failure, creating a vicious cycle. Premature ejaculation is a common psychosexual problem and responds well to the Acupressure Healing Program in Chapter 14.

Essential Dietary Considerations

For acupressure techniques to be effective in alleviating premature ejaculation, you must follow these dietary guidelines.

- Avoid foods containing large amounts of sugar or preservatives.
- Eliminate alcohol, drugs, and citrus juices from your diet.
- Give up coffee and all caffeinated drinks.
- Eat plenty of green vegetables, both raw and lightly cooked.
- Eat more fish, which contains the essential minerals for winning your battle.

Beans are a common Oriental folk remedy to benefit the reproductive organs. Adzuki beans are excellent for kidney disorders, while black beans are good for the sexual organs and a lack of sexual

Had we treated impotence as matter-of-factly as we treat a cold, there would probably be much less of it. A single incidence of temporary impotence can trigger a deep-seated fear of permanent impotence in a man.

—Akira Ishihara
and Howard Levy
The Tao of Sex

261

appetite. Eating a mixture of three parts grain to one part beans not only combines all the essential amino acids to make a complete protein but strengthens the reproductive system in both men and women. According to traditional Chinese medicine, an excess of sugar can imbalance the spleen, pancreas, and liver, which also taxes the kidneys. Avoid sugar, and eat a balanced diet of whole fresh foods.

In traditional Chinese eroticism, loveplay (what Westerners term foreplay) is not finished until a man has consciously touched his partner thoroughly all over and obtains four erection conditions: enlargement, engorgement, warmth, and hardness. Massaging a man's feet and toes can help him to obtain these four conditions of erection. The liver meridian originates in the large toe and governs the circulation of blood into the penis. Thus, stimulating the acupressure liver points on the thighs, feet, and toes can increase a man's sexual vitality.

Exploring Beyond the Genitals

A man may attain health and longevity if he practices an ejaculation frequency of twice monthly, or 24 times in a year. If at the same time he pays careful attention to proper diet and exercise, he will live a long and healthy life.

—Dr. Sun Ssu-Mo
Precious Recipes

A man's sexual vitality depends on the overall condition of his body, particularly his kidneys, liver, and prostate gland. In traditional Chinese medicine, the human body is an interconnected network of vital systems united by life energy, which is stored in the kidneys. When a man ejaculates excessively, he depletes this reserve energy and eventually his sexual vitality. (What constitutes excessive ejaculation varies among individuals, depending upon their physical strength, stamina, age, and even the season. Young men can ejaculate several times a week or even per day, while middle-aged and older men should conserve their more limited sexual energies and ejaculate only once or twice per week during the winter and perhaps two to three times per week in warmer months.) Thus, the condition of the kidneys governs potency: When the kidneys have an abundance of reserve energy, the male sexual-reproductive system is strong.

Losing control over what he thinks is his most important sexual tool is the greatest nightmare for many a man. In reality, his most important tool is his heart and his ability to use it to communicate his feelings, fears, and anxieties. Faced with premature ejaculation, he may avoid sex and blame his partner for not being thin enough or sexy enough. He may work excessively, become preoccupied with television shows or ball games, get drunk or stoned, or simply pick fights and blame his partner for creating an argument.

Incredible changes can happen, however, when a man at the bottom of his depression searches for an answer. If he explores Eastern sexology, he will find breathing exercises, dietary considerations, points to press, and a new perspective on making love. He will learn how to let go emotionally and discover new ways to use his penis. He will learn not only how to satisfy his partner when his penis is soft but how it can guide him to a deeper understanding of himself and his way of being with his partner.

Relieving Premature Ejaculation

During sexual arousal, the prostate gland becomes engorged with semen. When the prostate is weak, the fluid buildup creates the urgency to ejaculate prematurely. A man with sexual problems can treat himself naturally with his own male hormones by being careful not to ejaculate at all during intercourse. For maximum effectiveness, repeat this treatment several times a week. Fortunately, Taoist sexology offers these drug-free approaches for strengthening the prostate gland and relieving the pressures within it.

Deer Exercise

To gain greater ejaculatory control, practice this exercise regularly; it can be done anytime, anyplace. It is the same as the Kegel or "pelvic floor exercise" that doctors recommend to women who suffer from postdelivery urinary stress incontinence. Simply contract the muscles surrounding your anus while you simultaneously squeeze your genitals, as if you were stopping the flow of urine. Make the contractions strong and rhythmic, repeating them many times. Contract for 2 or 3 seconds, then relax for a couple of seconds. Repeat the contractions again and again—begin with three sets of 8 contractions. These contractions strengthen the prostate gland and slowly relieve the buildup of seminal fluid in the gland to gain ejaculatory control.

The Prostate's Potent Point

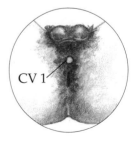

The acupressure point CV 1, located midway between the scrotum and rectum, can be helpful for coping with premature ejaculation. Feel for a slight indentation in this area. Press the point firmly for 2 minutes, which relieves pressure in the prostate and therefore the urgency to ejaculate prematurely. Pressing this point regularly on a daily basis for a couple of months can also strengthen the prostate gland. Your partner can participate by pressing this point for a few minutes before engaging in intercourse.

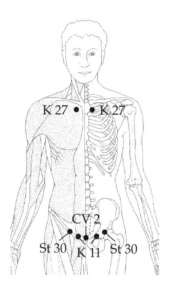

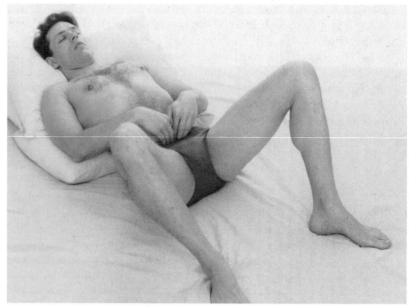

Ejaculation is always preceded by a rapid acceleration of the heart, thus you'll realize the importance of keeping your pulse normal during intercourse. Since breathing controls heartbeat, the first and foremost exercise for developing ejaculation control is deep, rhythmic abdominal breathing.

—Daniel P. Reid
*The Tao of Health,
Sex, and Longevity*

Rubbing Your Pubic Bone

Lie down on your back with your legs bent, feet flat on the floor or mattress. With the fingertips of both hands, briskly rub your pubic bone for about 90 seconds, 2 or 3 times a day. This acupressure massage on the pubic bone stimulates St 30, K 11, and CV 2. Follow it by rubbing the last point on the kidney meridian, K 27 (in the hollow below the head of the collarbones), for 1 minute to strengthen the male reproductive system.

Breath Control

When you feel yourself losing control of your ejaculation, take a deep swift inhalation into your lower abdomen, and hold your breath for 5 to 10 seconds. Roll your eyes back into your head. The combination of controlling the breath and rolling the eyes momentarily takes your mind away from your senses—long enough to regain ejaculatory control.

Tongue Touch

During intercourse, use the tip of your tongue to touch the back of the roof of your mouth. Move your tongue over the roof a couple of inches back until the hard palate becomes soft. When your tongue connects with the soft spot of the palate, as you breathe slowly and deeply, you can retain control and delay your ejaculation.

MISCELLANEOUS SEXUAL PROBLEMS

Primary acupressure points can be used to help overcome these other common difficulties relating to love and sex.

Vaginal Pain During Intercourse

Discomfort and pain during intercourse is a problem for many women. When it is not immediately dealt with, fears often become exacerbated and the problem can get worse. Explore the three following factors to deal with the root cause of the pain.

1. Medical Condition

First, see a doctor to determine whether you have a medical condition that is causing the pain. If your doctor doesn't find anything medically amiss with you, then it is appropriate to explore the next two factors.

2. Readiness

Pain during intercourse can be a natural signal that the body is not fully ready to be entered. Men typically move too fast toward intercourse. If intercourse occurs before the woman's body has had the time and stimulation to lubricate the walls of her vagina, it can be painful. Your partner must learn how to fully arouse you during foreplay. If your vagina does not fully moisten, have your partner use a natural lubricant. During and after menopause, women naturally produce less vaginal secretions; lubricants may also be helpful at this life stage.

3. Sexual Abuse or Inactivity

If you have been abused anytime in the past or if you have been sexually inactive for many months, you may need an especially patient partner and a much longer period of foreplay. When deep issues, concerns, and fears surface, the support of a body-oriented therapist can also be helpful.

Acupressure can relieve vaginal pain during intercourse provided that your partner uses sensitivity in gradually applying pressure. Use the lower back (B 23 and B 47) points with the central lower abdominal (CV 2–CV 6) points, as well as the Womb and Vitals (B 48) points and the groin points at Sp 12 and Sp 13. Hold each of these acupressure points with a firm supportive pressure for at least 2 minutes while you encourage your partner to breathe slowly and deeply into her belly.

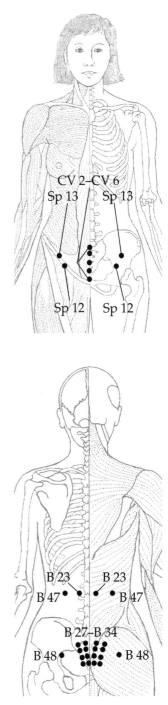

265

Painful or Tight Scrotum

A buildup of pressure in the scrotum, a common male symptom, can be extremely uncomfortable and disruptive in making love. This buildup can be due to various frustrations and blockages, or it can happen after having an erection, whether or not ejaculation occurs.

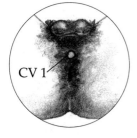

Holding the acupressure point between the rectum and genitals (CV 1) can relieve pain and pressure in the testicle area. When a man is resistant to being touched anywhere, especially in the genital region, there may be a buildup of fluids in the scrotum or prostate gland. Simply holding this acupressure point for 3 to 5 minutes can release the constriction and the associated pain.

To find the point, imagine a line between the anus and the center of the scrotum. CV 1 is located exactly midway between these two landmarks. When you press the correct point, you will find a soft spot. Use steady, firm pressure for about 5 minutes or until the pain subsides.

If the pain does not subside, remove your finger from the point. Contract and relax your anal and buttocks muscles thirty times in a heartbeat rhythm. Make the last five contractions strong.

Immediately apply finger pressure on the CV 1 point again, holding firmly without movement for 3 more minutes. End by holding the point gently for another minute. A blood pulsation at this point is a good sign, indicating increased circulation and relief.

Rectal Pain or Pressure

Another common sex-related complaint in both men and women is pressure in the anus. Holding two particular points can relieve this rectal pain.

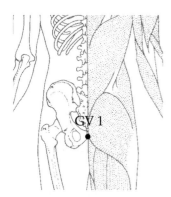

GV 1 is located under the tailbone. Place your middle finger underneath the tailbone, into the crack of the buttocks. Press upward and rub against the bottom of the tailbone, feeling for this sensitive spot.

The other acupressure point is CV 1, located directly between the anus and the genitals. When you find the correct point, you'll find a soft spot.

To relieve rectal pain, hold both of these points together for 3 to 5 minutes, until the pain diminishes.

Sexual Frustration

When sexual energy builds and isn't released, acupressure can be helpful for relaxation. Use the following five-step acupressure routine for relieving sexual frustration.

Have your partner lie down comfortably on his or her back.

1. Press the Groin

Place the palms of your hands on your partner's groin (Sp 12, Sp 13) where the tops of the legs join the trunk of the body. Adjust your hands to comfortably fit the shape of your partner's body, with your fingertips resting on the lower belly. Gradually lean some of your weight over your hands, directing the pressure into the lower abdomen. Have your partner breathe long, slow, deep breaths into the belly as you maintain the pressure in the groin for about 2 minutes.

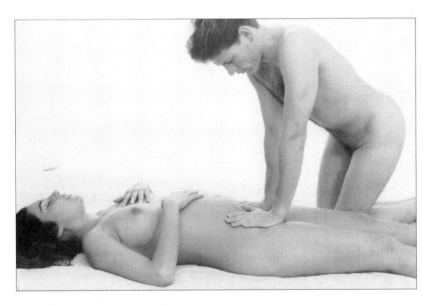

2. Chest-Belly Palming

Sit close to your partner's waist. Place the palm of one hand on the center of your partner's breastbone (CV 17) and the palm of your other hand in the center of your partner's lower belly, between the belly button and pubic bone (CV 4–CV 6). Encourage your partner to take slow deep breaths as you lightly rest your hands on your partner's body for 2 minutes.

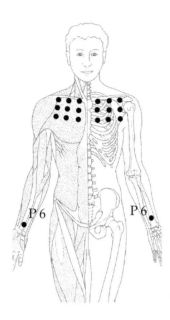

3. Chest Press

With your fingers, probe both sides of your partner's chest, feeling for any tightness below the collarbone. When you feel a tight spot, hold directly on it with light-to-firm pressure, depending upon your partner's preference. Hold both sides of the tightest muscles of the chest as you encourage your partner to breathe slowly and deeply into your finger pressure.

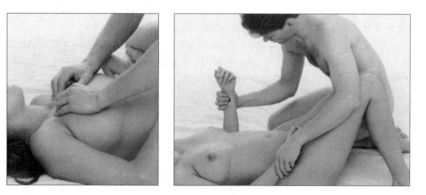

4. Squeeze Down the Arms

Use your hands on both sides to squeeze down the arm muscles from the shoulder to the Inner Gate (P 6). Hold these points on both sides with light pressure, using your thumbs, for 1 minute.

5. Finger Press

With your thumb and index finger, gently pull as you squeeze down the length of each finger, from the base to the nail. Do this for all ten fingers to move your partner's frustration out of his or her body.

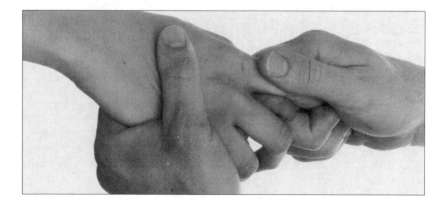

Chapter 14

ACUPRESSURE
HEALING PROGRAM

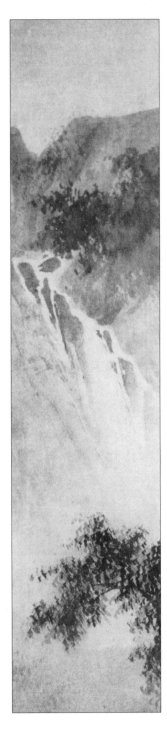

his Acupressure Healing Program has benefited many of the couples I have worked with, including some with deep-seated sexual problems. The program involves not having intercourse for at least a month to allow other aspects of sexual intimacy to develop without undue expectations. For example, after making great strides in overcoming their sexual problems and practicing the Acupressure Healing Routine three times a week for six weeks, Shelly and Bob (mentioned in Chapter 13) resumed having intercourse. Although it had taken discipline for them to abstain, they both felt afterward that this six-week period provided them with the safety to explore their sensuality and cultivate greater intimacy. It also gave Bob the confidence that once he lost an erection, he could regain it.

The Acupressure Healing Program, designed for both men and women, renews the body's sexual responsiveness. It is based on the vital components that sex therapists concur are essential for effective treatment of various sexual problems. All therapeutic work in this area owes a great deal to William Masters and Virginia Johnson, the pioneers who developed the first successful sexual therapy program.

The Acupressure Healing Program offers couples many opportunities to give and receive physical pleasure. They learn to feel the sexual experience in the whole body—not just genitally. Instead of depending on one pleasure center, couples have many pleasure centers, maximizing contact from head to toe. Acupressure's healing touch offers a greater understanding of how to relax, connect with each other, and increase your sexual energy.

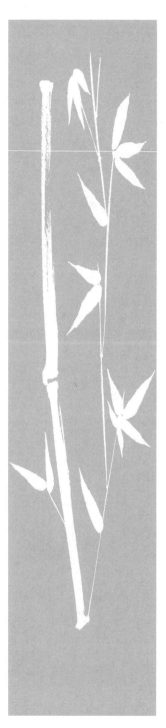

A HEALTHY LIFESTYLE

The Acupressure Healing Program requires you to choose a vigorous lifestyle, eat healthy foods, avoid excessive sugar, stretch your body, explore ways to reduce stress, and exercise daily. Consciously choosing what you eat and how much you exercise is your responsibility, not your partner's.

LETTING GO OF OLD ATTITUDES, EXPECTATIONS, AND DESTRUCTIVE PATTERNS

By releasing the muscular tensions that reinforce negative thoughts and judgments, acupressure provides couples with a positive way of relating to each other. Whether you knead each other's shoulders, exchange a back massage, or hold your partner's points while hugging or making love, the satisfying touch of acupressure can enable you to let go of your expectations and performance anxieties.

What is set in your mind is also embedded in your body. Thus, mental anxieties create corresponding tensions that inhibit sexual energy. As these tension patterns are released through acupressure, old attitudes, irritabilities, and frustrations begin to dissipate as well. While you make these mind-body changes, your acupressure points open further, and your life energy flows more and more strongly and freely.

The power of acupressure is cumulative: The more you do it, the better the results. What's more, as you give acupressure and enhance your partner's pleasure, you vicariously receive sexual energy and enjoyment. The giver doesn't control the experience and doesn't get drained.

Mutual care creates a perpetual healing cycle. When partners are giving the spirit of love through touch, a continuous flow of healing energy circulates through their points and meridians. The longer they practice mutual care, the more this vital energy generates a trusting, supportive, enduring relationship and deepens a truly sacred experience of sexuality.

ACUPRESSURE HEALING ROUTINE

This Acupressure Healing Routine consists of a series of three full-body couple's exercises, called Sensate Focus Exercises, designed to refocus your attention on sensations throughout your body and increase physical pleasure while reducing anxiety. In their program, Masters and Johnson forbade couples from having intercourse in the initial sessions, where refocus was being established. Thus, it is important to avoid touching the genitals until the male partner becomes comfortable with the experience of losing and regaining an erection. The Sensate Focus Exercises allow for increasing levels of stimulation, which after several weeks culminate in sexual intercourse.

These exercises have a number of vital purposes. . . .

They teach couples how to communicate:
- to take responsibility for sharing feelings and providing feedback without judgment, blame, shame, or guilt
- to express positive and negative emotions
- to verbalize their needs and desires for pleasure
- to give constructive criticism and direct requests without feeling shame or fear of hurting each other's feelings

They refocus couples' attention on sexual pleasure rather than the sex act:
- to increase relaxation and pleasure
- to remove performance pressures about intercourse
- to create a new definition of a good, satisfying sexual experience
- to encourage couples to set aside sacred time for developing physical intimacy in their relationship

They improve sexual orientation, function, and response:
- to increase the knowledge of each other's bodies
- to become more aware of the body and erogenous zones
- to develop a full sexual menu, enabling a couple to have a wide selection of playful appetizers, satisfying entrees, and exquisite desserts, including a variety of interesting postures and places to massage

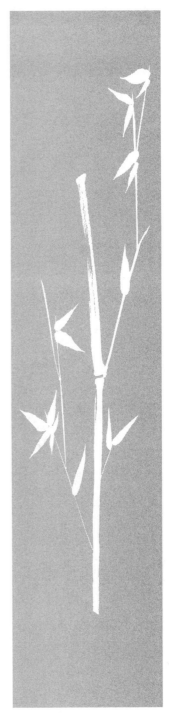

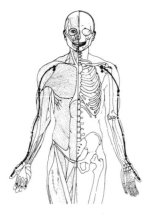

Lung Meridian

The Healing Routine, which is to be practiced daily, is based on the meridian pathways. Tracing these channels on each other's bodies paves the way for greater amounts of life energy to flow into the sexual reproductive system. Starting with the Lung and Large Intestine meridians, you will focus on breathing slowly and deeply together to gather the life force.

Be creative with your touch. Try new ways of stroking, caressing, and kneading the muscles. Ask your partner for feedback. Often women and men differ greatly in how they prefer to be touched. You may like a light touch, while your partner prefers firm contact. Accept the differences between you, encouraging your partner to guide you.

Enjoy letting go, and relax into the deep pleasure of being touched. Concentrate on breathing in and out together in sync throughout this massage. Guide your partner; give feedback on what feels good to you and what your body needs. Communicate clearly what works and what doesn't. Focus on your partner's sensual needs, and let go of achieving a sexual destination. Most of all, relax together and simply enjoy what is to come.

Part I: Touch and Be Touched

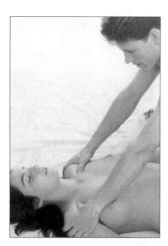

Caress, touch, and enjoy each other, avoiding genital and breast contact. If an erection occurs, do not take advantage of it. The purpose is to enjoy each other and learn what feels good, dethroning the idols of erection and intercourse, eliminating the pressure to perform in any way. In healthy relationships, the partners do not equate love with the sexual act. Try to practice this routine every day for at least one month.

Lung Meridian

The woman lies on her back, while the man sits comfortably at her side, his hips snug against her waist. Her arms stretch outward, her palms face up. The man traces the Lung meridian, placing his thumbs on the upper outer portion of her chest, with his fingertips rotated onto her shoulders. After taking several long, slow, deep breaths together, the man moves his hands from her chest down the arms to the thumbs. He leans toward her to apply firm pressure around the thumbs for about 5 seconds.

Large Intestine Meridian

Now the man traces the Large Intestine meridian on both sides. He begins by touching the tips of your partner's index fingers, slowly moving up along the outside of her arms to her shoulders. As he lightly kneads the shoulders, they both breathe deeply in sync. Then, he lightly caresses the outside of her neck, up to her face, ending on her cheek just beside her nose.

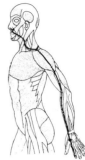

Large Intestine Meridian

Stomach Meridian

The man traces the Stomach meridian by continuing to caress the woman's face. They establish eye contact. He lightly glides his hands down over her throat, breasts, and groin, all the way down the outside of her legs, over the tops of her feet to the toes. By following this acupressure pathway, he touches many pleasurable places on his partner's body. Direct eye contact anchors this pathway, since the Stomach meridian begins at the eyes.

He follows this pathway with gentle loving kisses on the side of the throat, breasts, and nipples. As he moves through the abdominal muscles to the tip of the pubic bone, he seductively pauses. . . . From the tip of the pubic bone, he lightly traces the Stomach meridian down the outside of her legs over the tops of her feet to the large, ring, and middle toes. He massages her feet and toes thoroughly, spending extra time caressing the large toe.

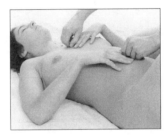

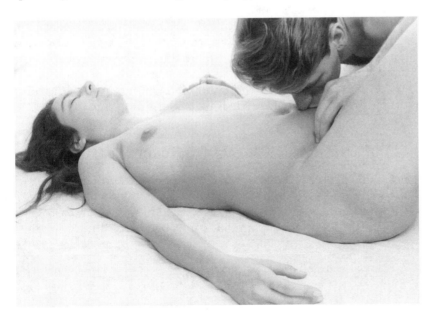

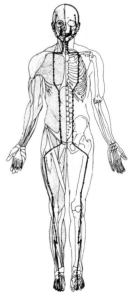

Stomach Meridian

273

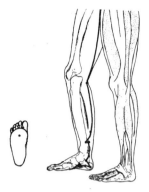

Kidney Meridian

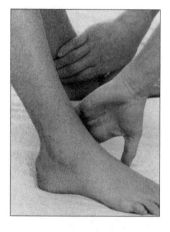

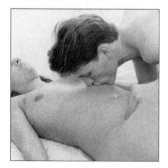

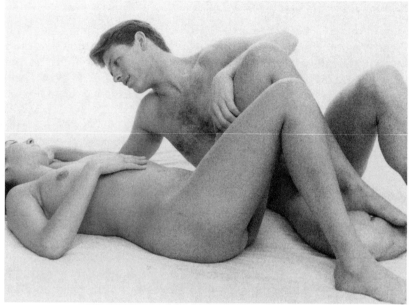

Kidney Meridian

To delight your partner sexually, work on the lower half of the Kidney meridian. Start by massaging the soles and arches of the feet, the insides of the heels and ankles. Then lightly glide your fingertips slowly up the insides of the legs toward your partner's genitals. The lighter you touch and the slower you move, the better. If you feel adventurous and want to spend more time with your partner, kiss, suck, and lick along the meridian, especially at each of the acupressure points. Making passionate sounds while breathing deeply on the Kidney meridian is particularly arousing.

Part II: Genital Touching Without Ejaculating

Let go of any expectations of having an orgasm during this part of the program. It will unfold naturally, in the fullness of time. Let it surprise you like a gift, something you didn't expect, a wonderful delight that cannot be planned, controlled, or willfully made to happen.

The man continues to stroke the Kidney meridian, beginning at the bottom of the feet, slowly caressing the insides of the woman's legs until she is so aroused that he too becomes turned on. He then takes hold of her hand and slowly lies down on his back beside her.

Her arousal draws her over him to reciprocate. She thoroughly stimulates each point on his Kidney meridian, starting at the bottom of his feet, paying special attention to the points around the ankle and up the inner thigh.

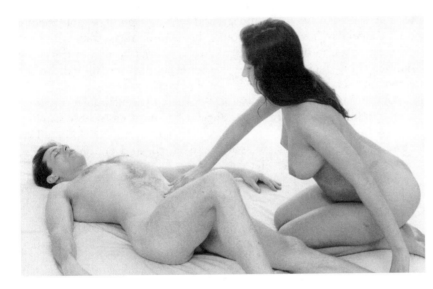

She gently caresses his scrotum and eventually his penis until he gets an erection. Then she stops touching his genital area until the erection goes away. She repeats this Sensate Focus Exercise several times to give the man practice getting, losing, and regaining an erection. She gazes into his eyes and breathes slowly and deeply each time she arouses him. He will learn that once his erection is lost, it can be revived.

The woman's middle fingertip settles into the CV 1 acupressure point, located directly between the anus and the genitals. She softly strokes the inner uppermost thigh, lightly caressing upward to bathe him with tantalizing, sensual ecstasy. Caress the hair between his buttocks and genitals. Once she comes close to the genitals, she takes her time gliding her hand slowly, very slowly. She watches her partner breathe and enjoys his pleasurable sounds and facial expressions.

Suck her nipples gently until they harden, and beyond, kissing her vulva and tickling her clitoris with your tongue until she is inundated with her own fluid between her thighs. Her arousal, in turn, will arouse you. Her excitement can give you an erection. If it does, then your problem is solved and you can enter her vagina easily.

—Jolan Chang
The Tao of Love and Sex

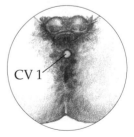

CV 1

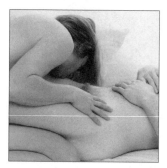

Part III: Intercourse

Practice Parts I and II daily for two weeks before engaging in Part III.

With the woman on top as the more active partner, the man can relax and does not have to feel obliged to make sexual intercourse happen. As she kisses, sucks, licks, and breathes on each point on the Kidney meridian, her hands are free to trace the meridian up the inside of his thighs toward his sexual organs. After lightly touching the hair underneath his scrotum, she presses the man's sacred point (CV 1), between his anus and genitals. At this point, if one partner doesn't feel like having intercourse, they simply relax, play with each other, or try one of the many positions in this book. On the other hand, if both feel like having intercourse, the woman can be the active partner on top, or they can be side by side.

Before engaging sexually, they agree to intentionally prolong intercourse. The female partner should be sensitive to withdrawing or slowing down when her partner comes close to ejaculating. This eliminates some of his pressure to perform and enables them to deeply relax and enjoy each other.

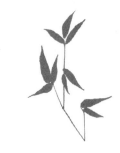

Man and woman should ebb and flow in intercourse like the waves and currents of the sea. In this manner, they may continue all night long, constantly nourishing and preserving their precious vital essence, curing all ailments, and promoting long life.

—Sun-Nu Ching
The Classic of the Plain Girl

I encourage you to continue practicing this full-body lovemaking routine, being present in the moment as you breathe fully and explore. The more you share your innermost selves—gazing into each other's eyes while touching and expressing the depths of your heart—the more your intimacy will become sacred. May this renewed intimacy be a celebration of your love—your hearts' total and uninhibited union. Enjoy loving each other as if it were the first time.

Appendix A

GENITAL REFLEXOLOGY

Over thousands of years of sexual exploration, the Chinese dicovered which positions stimulate specific genital areas, thus affecting certain health conditions, problems, and illnesses.

*Y*our whole body becomes revitalized when all the surfaces of your genitals are stimulated. A network of reflex points that correspond to all areas of the body are located on the penis and vagina, as on the feet and hands. Accordingly, excessively rubbing a specific area of your penis or vagina can overstimulate a corresponding organ, eventually resulting in various health problems. Genital areas corresponding to organs that do not get an adequate amount of stimulation may become energetically deficient and cause a dysfunction.

My Chinese sexology instructor, Dr. Stephen S. Chang, once told me about a case study that explains how valuable genital reflexology can be for sexually active couples. A married couple came to one of his associates' offices seeking help. The husband had suffered dramatic heart palpitations and thought he had experienced a heart attack. Several medical examinations and tests turned out to be negative, showing that nothing was wrong with his cardiovascular system. Dr. Chang's associate inquired of the couple what thay had been doing prior to the heart palpitations. They recalled that they were making love before the incident occurred. When asked to give specific details, the wife explained that she had been stimulating her husband with her mouth. When the sex counselor asked her how, she shyly described that she had used her tongue on the head of his penis, licking it like an ice cream cone. The sex counselor explained that the head of the penis corresponds with the heart. By sucking and licking the tip of his penis, she had overstimulated his heart.

When you touch or suck your partner's penis or vagina, you should give an equal amount of attention to the whole surface of the genital organ. Overstimulating one area can lead to problems. For instance, when a woman masturbates, the primary stimulation may be the clitoris, which corresponds to the kidneys and bladder. Excessive stimulation around the clitoris can tax the kidneys and possibly cause a bladder infection, water retention, or weight problems.

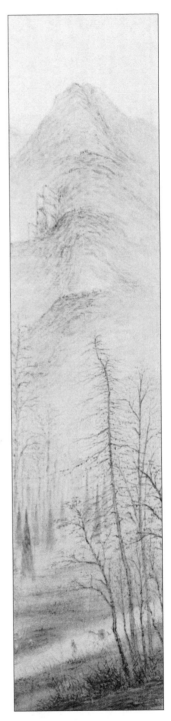

GENITAL REFLEXOLOGY

Heart

Lungs   Lungs

Uterus

Spleen
Pancreas

Cervix
Heart
Lungs

Liver

Spleen
Pancreas

Kidneys

Liver

Kidneys

Vaginal Opening

Zones of the Penis   **Zones of the Vagina**

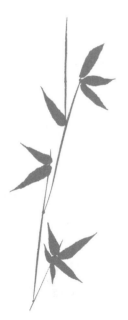

The reflexology zones in the vagina are mapped out the same as the penis, except in reverse order. Thus, when the penis fits snugly into the vagina, these reflex zones match, creating a powerful connection between both bodies. During intercourse, all of a man's and woman's genital reflex zones are in contact, creating one of the most pleasurable ways to heal all parts of the body.

Whether you stimulate your partner with your hand, mouth, or genitals, become aware of what parts of the sex organs are being most activated. Show each other new ways to stimulate the parts of the genitals that often get neglected. Explore new ways to touch the areas that often don't get attention. An awareness of genital reflexology encourages you to stimulate all parts of your sex organs for enhancing health, sexual fulfillment, and pleasure.

As you expand your awareness of the areas being stimulated and discover new positions that broaden your genital contact, all parts of your bodies benefit. As you experiment, you will find slight variations, such as bending your knees or placing a pillow underneath your hips, naturally changes the focus of your contact. Cultivating a variety of sexual positions can generate tremendous erotic energy for heightening your pleasures and vibrant health.

Appendix B

HEALTH BENEFITS OF
ACUPRESSURE FOR LOVE POINTS

Point	Name	Location	Benefit
GV 24.5	*Third Eye*	Directly between the eyebrows, in the indentation where the bridge of the nose meets the forehead	Balances the pituitary gland; also relieves hot flashes, hay fever, sinus pain, headache, and general stress.
CV 17	*Sea of Tranquility*	On the center of the breastbone, four finger-widths up from the base of the breastbone, in an indentation	Relieves nervousness, anxiety, hypertension, anguish, depression, and other emotional imbalances
GB 21	*Shoulder Well*	On the highest point of the top of the shoulder muscle, one inch out from the base of the lower neck	Relieves fatigue, shoulder tension, poor circulation, nervous problems, and stiff necks
TW 15	*Heavenly Rejuvenation*	On the shoulder muscles, one-half inch directly below GB 21	Balances body temperature, relieves shoulder pain, poor circulation, and fatigue
GV 20	*One Hundred Meeting*	Place your fingers behind your ears. Move your fingertips up to the top of your head, feeling for a hollow toward the back of the center of the top of the head	Relieves headache, sinus problems, weak sense of smell, insomnia, epilepsy, high blood pressure, heat stroke, hot flashes, and vertigo; good for memory and concentration
GV 21	*Anterior Summit*	One thumb's width in front of GV 20	Same as GV 20

Point	Name	Location	Benefit
GV 19	*Posterior Summit*	One thumb's width in back of GV 20	Same as GV 20
B 7	*Penetrating Heaven*	On top of the skull one thumb's width from the center, in line with the back of the ears	Relieves headache, stuffy nose, insomnia, and head congestion
H 7	*Spirit Gate*	On the little finger side of the forearm, at the crease of the wrist	Relieves insomnia, anxiety, hypertension, forgetfulness, and calms the spirit
GB 20	*Gates of Consciousness*	Below the base of the skull, in the hollows two to three inches apart depending on the size of the head	Relieves depression, insomnia, headache, dizziness, stiff neck, shoulder pain, uptightness, and irritability
GV 16	*Wind Mansion*	In the center of the back of the head, in the large hollow under the base of the skull	Relieves headache, stiff neck, neck pain, dizziness, hyper-tension, influenza, and colds
B 10	*Heavenly Pillar*	One finger-width below the base of the skull on the ropy muscles and one-half inch out from the spine	Relieves stress, overexhaus-tion, insomnia, heaviness in the head, eyestrain, stiff neck, and sore throats
B 23 and B 47	*Sea of Vitality*	In the lower back two (B 23) and four (B 47) finger-widths from the spine at waist level	Relieves depression, high blood pressure, trauma, lower backache, chronic fatigue, and sexual-reproductive problems
B 48	*Womb and Vitals*	Two finger-widths outside the sacrum (at the base of the spine)	Relieves pelvic tension, hip pain, PMS, lower backache, sciatica, menstrual cramps, and general frustrations
B 27–B 34	*Sacral Points*	On the base of the spine, in the hollows of the bone	Relieves hip pain, sacral pain, lower back pain, and sciatica

Point	Name	Location	Benefit
GB 14	*Yang White*	On the forehead, one finger-width above the eyebrows, directly up above the pupil	Relieves eyestrain, head congestion, mental stress, headache, and eye twitch
B 2	*Drilling Bamboo*	In the indentation of the eye socket, where the nose bridge meets the eyebrow ridge	Relieves sinus pain, headache, blurry vision, red and watery eyes, hay fever, and eyestrain
K 27	*Elegant Mansion*	In the depression directly below the protrusions of the collarbone	Relieves breathing difficulties, asthma, sore throat, coughing, and depression
K 3	*Bigger Stream*	In the back of the ankle, between the inside ankle-bone and Achilles tendon	Relieves sexual problems, swollen feet, back pain, ankle pain, and fatigue
Sp 4	*Grandparent-Grandchild*	In the upper arch of the foot, one thumb-width from the ball of the foot	Relieves foot cramps, PMS, bloating, and indigestion
P 1	*Heavenly Pond*	One thumb-width outside the nipple	Relieves breast and chest pain and swollen lymph glands
St 16	*Breast Window*	Above the breast tissue in line with the nipples	Relieves breast pain, lactation problems, and heartburn
St 17	*Center of the Breasts*	In the center of the nipple	Opens sensual experiences
Sp 12 Sp 13	*Rushing Door Mansion Cottage*	In the middle of the crease where the leg joins the trunk of the body	Relieves menstrual cramps, abdominal discomfort, and reproductive problems
CV 4– CV 6	*Sea of Intimacy*	Two and four finger-widths below the navel	Relieves PMS, impotence, and uro-reproductive problems
CV 24	*Supporting Nourishment*	Midway between the center of the lower lip and chin	Increases intimacy and genital pleasures

Point	Name	Location	Benefit
CV 1	*Inner Meeting*	At the center of the perineum, midway between the anus and genitals	Relieves pressure in the genitals and rectum, hemorrhoids, impotence, prostate problems, and premature ejaculation
CV 2	*Crooked Bone*	On the top of the public bone in the center	Benefits the reproductive system and bladder
K 11	*Transverse Bone*	One-half finger-width from the midline, on the upper border of the pubic bone	Relieves impotence, lower abdominal pain, scrotum pain, and urinary problems
K 1	*Bubbling Spring*	On the center of the sole of the foot, at the base of the ball of the foot, between the two pads	Relieves hot flashes, infertility and impotence; a first-aid revival point
Lv 10–Lv 12	*Inner Thigh*	On the inside of the upper thigh, close to the inner crease where the thigh joins the trunk of the body	Relieves infertility, genital pains, gynecological disorders, and cold feet; increases sexual energy
Sp 6	*Three Yin Meeting*	Four finger-widths above the inside anklebone, on the back border of the shinbone	Relieves menstrual cramps, vaginal discharge, genital pain, and water retention
B 13–B 15 and B 36–B 38	*Emotional Support*	Between the shoulder blades and the spine, at the level of the heart and lungs	Relieves hypertension, high blood pressure, and insomnia; calms the spirit
Lu 1	*Letting Go*	On the outer upper chest, four finger-widths up from the armpit crease and one finger-width inward	Relieves depression, shallow breathing, coughing, asthma, and skin disorders; strengthens the lungs
P 5 P 6	*Intermediary Inner Gate*	Three and four finger-widths above the center of the inner wrist crease, between the tendons	Relieves upset stomach, nausea, morning sickness, indigestion, and wrist pain; balances the emotions

OTHER WORKS BY THE AUTHOR*

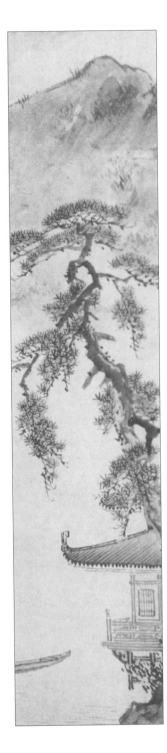

ACUPRESSURE VIDEOS FOR COUPLES*

- Acupressure for Lovers: The Video
  Enhancing Sexual Intimacy
- Embracing Love: Acupressure for Sacred Sexuality
- Joy for Lovers: Music and Movements to Open the Heart

ACUPRESSURE POINT REFERENCE CHART

24" x 36" full-color laminated poster
Front, back, and side views—in one chart
Includes point recipe booklet for common ailments

ACU-YOGA VIDEOS*

- For Stress Relief
- For Flexibility: Stretches for Long Life
- For Meridians: Daily Self-Care Exercises

ARTHRITIS RELIEF AUDIOTAPTES

- Tape 1: *Morning & Evening Routines*
- Tape 2: *Self-Acupressure Techniques*
- Tape 3: *Self-Care for Relieving Hand Pain*

BOOKS

- Acupressure's Potent Points: *Relieving Common Ailments*
- Arthritis Relief at Your Fingertips: *Self-Care for Joint Pain*
- Greater Energy at Your Fingertips: *10 Minutes to Vitality*
- Acu-Yoga: *Self-Help Techniques to Relieve Tension*
- The Bum Back Book: *Acupressure Self-Help Back Care*

* For further information on these instructional resources contact:
Acupressure Institute, 1533 Shattuck Ave., Berkeley, CA 94709,
(800) 442-2232 or (510) 845-1059 in California.

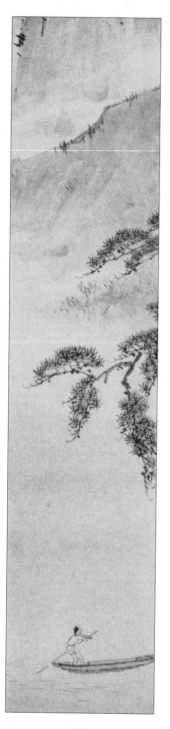

AUDIOTAPES FOR WOMEN

- Weight Loss: *Decrease Hunger & Fatigue*
- PMS Relief: *Relieve Menstrual Discomfort or Cramps*
- Greater Beauty: *Enjoy a Natural, Non-surgical Facelift*
- Techniques for Greater Energy: *Revitalize Yourself!*

REFRESHER AUDIOTAPES

- The 5:00 Refresher: *Revitalize Yourself after Work*
- The Traveler's Refresher: *You'll Arrive Feeling Great!*
- The Smoker's Refresher: *Extra Energy to Break the Habit*
- The Rush Hour Refresher: *Relieve Stress While You Drive*
- Acu-Yoga Audio Course: Contains 5 cassettes & booklet

INSTRUCTIONAL ACUPRESSURE VIDEOS*

- Fundamentals of Acupressure Video
- Releasing Shoulder and Neck Tension
- Bum Back Video: *Self-care Back Exercises and Acupressure*
- Zen Shiatsu Video: *Instruction for Aspiring Practitioners*

HANDS-ON INSTRUCTIONAL BOOKLETS

- Acu-Face Lift: *A Beauty Workbook*
- Acupressure Weight Loss: *Points, Exercises and Recipes*
- Acupressure for Health Professionals
- Basic Acupressure: *Points and Channels*
- Hand and Foot Reflexology
- Introduction to Acupressure Booklet
- Traditional Chinese Dietary Therapy

For more information on these healing books, tapes, and videos request the mail order *Hands-On Health Care Catalog* by calling the phone number below.

* Order any three assorted video programs listed on pages 283-284 and receive $10 off the regular price. Order four or more assorted videotapes and get $20 off the regular price.

—Mastercard and Visa accepted—
Call **(800) 442-2232** or **(510) 845-1059** in California.

RESOURCES:
FOR GOING FURTHER

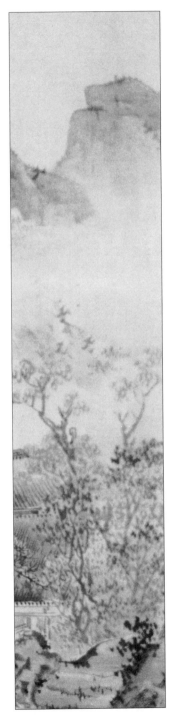

Acupressure Training

Since 1976, the Acupressure Institute in Berkeley, California, has offered year-round career training programs in Asian bodywork and therapeutic massage. These trainings are approved by the California Department of Education and the Board of Registered Nurses. Basic training (150 hours) includes hands-on instruction in acupressure massage, shiatsu techniques, Jin Shin style, more than 75 acupressure points, five elements theory, pulse reading, dietary principles, reflexology, and anatomy. After the training, small group apprenticeship follow-ups are also offered.

Intensive Trainings

The Acupressure Institute also offers popular one-month basic trainings five times a year in the San Francisco Bay Area. This program is also offered every spring in Minneapolis, Minnesota, and each fall on the East Coast as four extensive weekend workshops. To receive a complete course catalog, an application for admission, and a current schedule of classes, call the Acupressure Institute toll-free at (800) 442-2232 or (510) 845-1059. A list of housing resources is available for out-of-town students taking the training in Berkeley.

Acupressure Workshops

Michael Reed Gach, Ph.D., personally teaches couple's workshops and acupressure throughout the world. Write to the Acupressure Institute about organizing a weekend workshop in your area, including your date preferences (allow at least ten months lead time), your phone number, and the best times to reach you. Choose which workshop you would like to sponsor: "Acupressure for Relieving Common Complaints" or "Acupressure for Lovers."

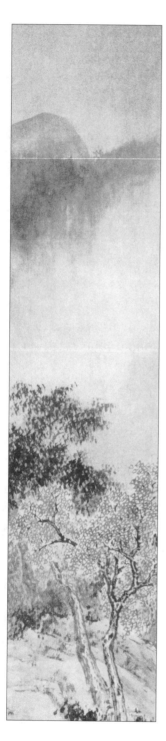

Videos for Lovers

Experience the flow of the hands-on acupressure techniques described in this book, sensitively narrated by the author, Michael Reed Gach. Each video presents how to stimulate your partner's acupressure points while embracing and making love for increased intimacy and pleasure. These erotic programs for couples, like exercise videos, are designed to be used again and again to practice. Each instructional video provides the movements, timing and guidance to make this book come alive with your partner. Call or write the Acupressure Institute for more information.

Hands-On Health Care Catalog

The Acupressure Institute distributes a wide variety of educational and self-care books, charts, flash cards, and instructional videotapes. You will find hands-on health care products that can support your personal healing, show you how to use acupressure to relieve common ailments, and enhance your life. Call or write to receive a free copy of *Hands-On Health Care*, the Acupressure Institute's mail-order catalog:

Acupressure Institute 1533 Shattuck Ave. Berkeley, CA 94709
(800) 442-2232 (outside CA) • (510) 845-1059 (in CA)

National Practitioner Directory

The American Oriental Bodywork Therapy Association (AOBTA) publishes an annual directory of teachers and practitioners of Oriental bodywork. For a quarterly newsletter, information on annual conferences, or a practitioner directory, contact:

AOBTA 1000 White House Rd. Suite 510 Voorhees, NJ 08043
(609) 782-1616 • (609) 782-1653 Fax

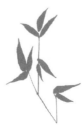

ACKNOWLEDGMENTS

My roots and values for quality human relationships stem from my dear parents. Through their consistent, unconditional love, I have always had an ease in expressing my heart and creating intimacy. I am blessed to have parents who trust themselves and love me with all their hearts.

Susan Graff Mills greatly inspired me while I wrote this book. She conceived of the idea of creating the Lovemaking Progressions, offering couples a series of erotic activities from greeting to making love. Patricia Lynn Reilly skillfully outlined some of the chapters, provided the initial research and sparked my own writing. I recommend readers look for her books and tapes on women's spirituality. I am also grateful to my long-time, dear friend Vivianna Watson who reviewed and critiqued all the love positions with me. Vivianna's experience in the Tantric healing arts was a valuable contribution to the book.

I want to thank Janett Blondeau and Joella Caskey who transcribed the entire manuscript. I appreciated Janett's editing and organizational skills, which kept the manuscript together as a whole. In terms of design, I'd like to thank Mary Sanichas and Karin Kinsey for their creative desktop publishing expertise and their graphic input in shaping the book's design. I also want to acknowledge Anca Sira for her artistic illustrations. Once again, I enjoyed working with David Lehrer, who shot all of the fine photography. Finally, I'd like to express appreciation for the couple who gave me the most feedback as my guinea lovers: Wendy Barry and Richard Owen.

In terms of editorial guidance, Leslie Meredith and Mark Mayell deserve to be acknowledged for their literary talent, clarity, and vision. They helped me more than anyone to shape the structure and tone of this book. I am also grateful for the editorial assistance I received from my mother, Julie Shpiesel, Brian Tart, Candace Coar, Linda Gross, and Andrea Epel. I want to thank my friends and teachers at the Acupressure Institute for their support and professional suggestions, especially Joseph Carter, L.Ac., and Alice Hiatt, R.N.

I photographed all the nature shots that open each chapter and painted the bamboo. I am responsible for how each page looks. Most authors are not given that role. I directed all the photography, typography, graphics, book design, and page layouts.

I feel blessed to have teachers who enriched my life and greatly contributed to this book. Zobra Kalinkowitz taught me the art of Oriental brush painting, its philosophy, basic practices, and the Zen of seeing nature. In Maui, Michael Eisenberg taught me the Thai massage stretches in Chapter 11. I appreciate the clarity, depth, and spirit of both Michael's and Zohra's teaching. Dr. Stephan Chang first introduced me to the ancient art of Chinese sexology over fifteen years ago. In studying Tantra, I learned most from Charles and Carolyn Muir and Daniel Reid's books. I am also grateful for studying point location and point therapeutics with Dr. Frank Chung, L.Ac., O.M.D. I will always love these teachers.

INDEX

ABOUT THE AUTHOR

Michael Reed Gach, Ph.D., is an authority on acupressure therapy for both self-treatment and alternative health care. Michael is the founder of the Acupressure Institute's bodywork school, located in Berkeley, California. Dr. Gach's groundbreaking natural techniques— the result of more than 25 years of in-depth study—have brought healing to thousands. He is the author of *Acu-Yoga, Acupressure's Potent Points, Greater Energy at Your Fingertips, The Bum Back Book,* and *Arthritis Relief at Your Fingertips.*

Dr. Gach produced an instructional series of *Acupressure for Lovers Videotapes* based on his book. He also created many other instructional videotapes for home study, such as *Fundamentals of Acupressure, Zen Shiatsu,* and *Acu-Yoga Stress Relief.* Dr. Gach designed the full-color *Acupressure Point Reference Chart* and its companion booklet showing which points to use for common complaints. Michael also teaches workshops for couples and conducts acupressure trainings throughout the world.

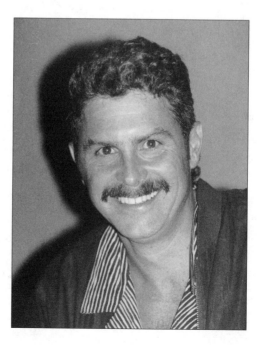